Values in Professional Practice: lessons for health, social care and other professionals

Edited by

Stephen Pattison

School of Religious and Theological Studies, Cardiff University

and

Roisin Pill

School of General Practice Cardiff University

RADCLIFFE MEDICAL PRESS

OXFORD · SAN FRANCISCO

Radcliffe Publishing Ltd
18 Marcham Road
Abingdon
Oxon OX14 1AA
United Kingdom

www.radcliffe-oxford.com
Electronic catalogue and worldwide online ordering.

_____

British Library Cataloguing in Publication Data

A catalogue record for this book is available from the British Library.

ISBN 1 85775 818 8

Typeset by Acorn Bookwork, Salisbury, Wiltshire
Printed and bound by TJ International Ltd, Padstow, Cornwall

Contents

Foreword

The central message in this book is that a 'static uncritical view of professions and values is simply not tenable in contemporary society and social institutions'. The implication is that researchers, policymakers, members of organisations, professional legislators, educators and trainers, individual professionals and workers or users of the service of professions and professionals need to take more seriously the dynamic, conflicting and changing relationships which form the living ecology surrounding values and professions today.

Values in Professional Practice: lessons for health, social care and other professionals is, in part, the outcome of a workshop which was held at the Nuffield Trust. We were delighted to support this initiative because we believe these issues matter, and will continue to matter, very much. The Nuffield Trust is perhaps best known for its concerns with health, healthcare, and management, so many of the chapters herein are centrally relevant to its concerns. However, the Trust also tries to engender innovation and discussion in all parts of society and in a wide variety of professional groups and organisations. As many of the contributions to this book show, values cannot be the province of any one profession, organisation, or group. Healthcare and other organisations and professions are part of a wider value ecology which helps to shape them. It is very much in the interests of society as a whole that much wider understanding and debate is engendered about the place of values throughout a variety of occupations and groups.

As a former healthcare manager, I am all too aware of the vital importance of value consonance and dissonance in any kind of organisation. An example of self-defeating value dissonance springs readily to mind. To improve their competitive position, SAS (Scandinavian Airlines) adopted the concept of the learning organisation, empowering staff at all levels. Unfortunately, the airline forgot that it was crucial to have Main Board endorsement of the organisation's values. This should be a critical part of organisation design and the economic consequences of getting it wrong were severe.

The Board decided to focus on the more profitable business-class customers but instead SAS became one of the most popular airlines with economy-class passengers, whose numbers increased while business-class numbers declined to such an extent that it put the airline at risk. The reason was simple. SAS employees, with their very egalitarian Scandinavian outlook, arrived at their own interpretation of the values of the business. Check-in staff saw that the business-class traveller had a great many comforts and advantages which were denied to the economy passenger and they decided to focus their customer care efforts on the economy-class passengers. It wasn't long before it was realised that the Board had to agree values – they cannot be generated by individual staff at their own discretion.

It is not just in private companies or at the level of organisational policy that values make an important contribution to the feel and competence of professional work. Anyone who has had to work in an environment in which they feel their own personal values clash with those of the organisation will know how painful and dysfunctional this can be both for themselves and others around them. One of the main contributions that this book might make is to provide readers from many different backgrounds – professional, personal and organisational – with a vocabulary with which to begin to articulate the importance, ambivalence and discomforts that can surround the enactment of values in the turbulent environment surrounding professions of all kinds today.

The editors of this book assert that 'values are everybody's business'. It is my belief that readers will become convinced of the veracity of this assertion once they have read the fascinating and very varied discussions of the ways in which values and professions have interacted, and continue to interact.

John Wyn Owen CB
Secretary
The Nuffield Trust
London
March 2004

Acknowledgements

The book before you is a joint production. Most of the chapters in it have been written by an interdisciplinary group of researchers and practitioners interested, from a variety of perspectives, in values in professional practice. The group's core membership is based around South Wales and the South West of England. One member who has not contributed in writing here is Patricia Lyne of the University of Wales College of Medicine.

The group has been fortunate not only in its pluriform local membership but also in its more distant friends. We would particularly like to thank James Armstrong, Eileen Fegan, Stephen Howell and Jeremy Roche for contributing chapters to this volume.

Beyond the writers of chapters herein are a group of people from a variety of disciplines who kindly attended a symposium at the Nuffield Trust, London in 2002 to discuss the drafts and themes that have led to this book. Many thanks to Iona Heath (general practitioner), Hilary Scott (deputy National Health Service Ombudsman), Jerry Bingham (UK Sport), Nicola Walsh (management academic), Phil George (journalist and producer), Madeleine Bidder (lawyer), Ruth Adams (Royal Society of Arts), Stephen Crow (planner) and Annabelle Mark (management academic) for giving so much time and enthusiasm to this project. On behalf of the group, we would particularly like to record thanks to the Nuffield Trust and its chief executive, John Wyn Owen, for supporting this venture in such a helpful way and at such a crucial time in its development.

As editors, we would like to thank the authors of the chapters in this book for working to time and submitting drafts and corrections speedily, efficiently and without complaint or excuse. It is an unusual and enjoyable privilege to work with such a friendly, co-operative group of people in addition to working on such interesting subject matter in the chapters themselves. This speaks highly of the sense of commitment that has built up in the pursuit of understanding values in professional practice. In this context, we would like to thank the values in professional practice core group for entrusting us with editing this book, together with draconian powers for ensuring it was produced. It is a tribute to our colleagues that we never had to resort to the latter!

Gillian Nineham and her colleagues at Radcliffe Medical Press have been exemplary in their enthusiasm for the book and their competence in ensuring its eventual publication.

It only remains to hope that readers of this book will find it as enjoyable to read as we have found it to produce. We would welcome feedback, comments, suggestions and more collaborators as we move forward as a group to research more aspects of the fascinating topic of values in professional practice. If you would like to enter into dialogue with us, please contact Stephen Pattison (PattisonS@Cardiff.ac.uk).

Stephen Pattison
Roisin Pill
March 2004

About the editors

Stephen Pattison is Head of the School of Religious and Theological Studies at Cardiff University. A member of the ethics committee of the Royal College of General Practitioners, he has been a healthcare chaplain and a National Health Service manager.

Roisin Pill is a professor in the School of General Practice, Cardiff University, and has published on health service research and medical sociology topics. She has also been vice chair of a health authority and chaired a local research ethics committee.

About the contributors

James Armstrong was an engineering consultant. He was President of the Institution of Structural Engineers in 1989/90 and a member of a review panel redrafting the Code of Practice for the Institution of Civil Engineers.

Paul Ballard is a professor at the School of Religious and Theological Studies, Cardiff University. He specialises in practical theology with an emphasis on the social context of British religion.

Andrew Edgar is a senior lecturer in philosophy at Cardiff University. He is Director of the Cardiff Centre for Applied Ethics and the author of numerous articles on medical ethics and aesthetics.

Eileen V Fegan is a lecturer in law at Queen's University, Belfast. She has held positions at Lancaster, Oxford and Cardiff universities and specialises in legal education, jurisprudence and feminist theory.

Ben Hannigan is a senior lecturer in mental health nursing at the School of Nursing and Midwifery Studies, Cardiff University. His practitioner background is in community mental health nursing.

Stephen Howell is Head of Leisure Services at Derwentside District Council with responsibility for sport, arts and outdoor services. He has been influential in the development of a number of new sport and leisure facilities and heads a sports development service.

Michael McNamee is a senior lecturer in philosophy at the Centre for Philosophy, Humanities and Law in Healthcare, University of Wales, Swansea. He has edited books on the ethics of leisure, sport and research and on the philosophy of science in exercise, health and sport research.

Jeremy Roche is Director of the Health and Social Care Programme at the School of Health and Social Welfare at the Open University. He has written widely on social work and the law and in the 1990s was on the management committee of the Children's Legal Centre.

Huw Thomas is a reader in the School of City and Regional Planning, Cardiff University. He has been a planner with a local authority, and has also been convenor of the equal opportunities (race relations) panel of the Royal Town Planning Institute.

Paul Wainwright is a reader in humanities and healthcare and Joint Head of the Centre for Philosophy, Humanities and Law in Healthcare at the University of Wales, Swansea. He has worked as a nurse in the NHS and as a professional advisor to a nursing statutory body.

Andrew Wall is a visiting senior fellow at the Health Services Management Centre, University of Birmingham. For 18 years he held the most senior managerial post in the Bath Health District.

Introduction

This book should be of interest to anyone who is involved with or affected by professions and their activities. That probably means everyone. Many readers will be professionals. All of us are affected on a daily basis by the work that professionals do. We have become dependent upon the professions in every significant area of life. We cannot be born, become educated, get married, have children, be sick, be well, manage our financial affairs, plan and build our houses, buy and dispose of property, govern and be governed, die or be buried without the aid of professionals. Crucially, to be involved in a profession, or to benefit from professional activity, is to be affected by, and to engage with, its values, either directly or indirectly.

There are few areas of contemporary life which do not involve professional activity and the values that inform it. Strangely, while values are much talked about, they are relatively little examined or critically understood in professions today. Values are a familiar concept and an integral part of professional life, manifesting themselves in charters, oaths, codes of practice, mission statements and different kinds of individual and occupational behaviour. However, few people seem to understand what values are, how they are constructed, or how they function in anything but the most general sense (New 2002). Nor does there seem to be very much active curiosity as to how they function specifically in professional life, in different kinds of professions and in different contexts. The relationship between ethics and professions has received some interest and coverage (Koehn 1994) and specific ethical issues more, but the relationships between fundamental values and professional practice have been ignored.

There is little understanding of how values inform or affect actual practices for individuals or institutions. Similarly, there is not much interest in understanding how experience and practice may mould or transform values in particular situations. For the most part, professionals and their clients seem content to assume that the values they have are the right ones and that there is little that can be done to advance, change or understand them. Furthermore, there is not much interest in whether other professions share the same values or adopt ones that fundamentally conflict.

The aim of this book is to break the uncritical silence about the relationship between values and professions and to provide a critical introduction to the ways in which values are understood by, and impinge upon, different professional groups. We hope it will contribute to a better informed, more critical discussion of the place of values in professional life and practice, as well as suggesting ways in which values can be more effectively articulated and researched.

Issues, questions and themes that pertain to this discussion will emerge as the book progresses. However, it is pertinent here to indicate the significance of studying values in professional practice in a preliminary way and to provide a taster of what is to come.

The importance of studying values and professional practice

Values and professional practice are basically everybody's business. More than this, the consideration of the relationship between these two elements opens up issues that raise fundamental theoretical and practical questions about the nature of professionals, professions and values. Here are just a few examples of the sorts of issues that are raised. These will be developed and supplemented as the book progresses.

Professional identity

Values are a key part of professional identity, helping to orient professionals as a group and to distinguish occupational groups from each other. So how do professions evolve, sustain and change their values over time? Are there common values that all professions should espouse and maintain? Can similar or common values apply to different professional groups so that architects or sportspeople can basically sign up to the same values as members of caring professions like doctors, nurses and physiotherapists? Or do different values apply to different professions?

The nature of professions in society

Many workers and occupational groups in contemporary society aspire to be designated as professional, despite the fact that professions and their members are often regarded with a certain amount of suspicion by their clients. (George Bernard Shaw's epithet in the Preface to *The Doctor's Dilemma* about professions being 'conspiracies against the laity' is much quoted in this context [Shaw 1946].) To ask questions about values in this context is to ask fundamental questions about the nature and position of professions in their social context. At issue in much of the discussion of values is the fundamental notion of trust (O'Neill 2002). What values can we expect professions and professionals to subscribe to in theory and enact in their practice? Whose values do they serve? How are these values policed and reproduced? Can anyone change them? Or are they (and we) stuck with them forever?

Formation and practice

Issues of professional identity and context lead naturally to consideration of how individuals are to relate their own values to the demands of the occupational groups that they join, and how they are moulded into the values and expectations of peers and colleagues. The relationship between the 'naïve' personal values of professional initiates, and how these are or should be shaped and changed as they are trained for a particular role, is not one that has received the attention it deserves. Should professional trainees leave their own values at the door of the classroom or the workplace? What should they do when they experience the pain of fundamental value conflict? How might individuals interpret and enact the values of occupational groups as expressed in codes or charters, particularly if there are conflicts between them? And how might teachers, trainers and professional bodies help their members to become more competent mediators and interpreters of professional values in practice?

The nature of values themselves

The consideration of professional practice brings into question the nature of values themselves. What, in fact, are the values that commend themselves to professionals? Are there different kinds of values that influence professionals? Are there, for example, non-moral values that affect practice as much as ethical values and principles? Are the fine theoretical 'motherhood and apple pie' values such as justice, honesty and transparency that adorn formal professional utterances the ones that are enacted in everyday life? And what is the relationship between any different categories and types of values that come into play in professional life?

These issues and others are raised in the chapters that follow. They are far from academic, as readers will see. They require far more critical attention than they have hitherto received.

The nature of this book and how to use it

The chapters herein have been written by an interdisciplinary authorship from many different academic and practice backgrounds – from philosophy to leisure services – with a heavy input from those concerned with health and caring professions in between. This diverse authorship will allow readers to examine a range of professions from a variety of disciplinary perspectives that will throw light on the pluriform nature of professions, professionals and the ways that they relate to their own and others' values. The range of professions and analytic perspectives provided will enable readers to see the overlaps and differences, the gaps and uniting themes, that emerge in considering professional values today. Those who persist to the end of the book, reading all or most of it, will develop a clear and fascinating overview of how different professions and professionals might conceive of, handle, and be affected by the values they adopt.

While we believe that all those who have anything to do with professions and professionals will find substantial matter here to interest them, the book will be of particular relevance to some specific audiences. Individual professionals in all professional groups should be able to find much here that will help them to reflect critically on the place of values in their own everyday practice. Those who organise and legislate for particular professions, creating charters, codes of practice and so on, will find many of the chapters of direct use in trying to develop critical horizons and practice. Similarly, educators for the professions and their students will discover a useful range of perspectives and insights that will stimulate thought and debate in the classroom and beyond. Last, but not least, we hope that academic researchers whose work relates to professional practice will find this a stimulating source of ideas and methods for taking much needed debate further.

This is neither a handbook nor a textbook: it is far from comprehensive. Interdisciplinary enquiry into professions and values is not well developed. So this volume is really a starting point, a source of questions and ideas that need to be explored in much further depth.

That said, we try, throughout the book in the individual chapters and particularly in editorial introductions to the five parts, to summarise common emergent themes, issues and questions. All the authors of the book have met each other on several occasions to discuss their contributions. So it is to be hoped that the work transcends simply being a collection of disparate papers held together only with the concepts of professions and values.

We very much hope that many readers will want to read this book from beginning to end. Only by doing this will it become clear how rich a topic this is, how divergent approaches and practices are in different professional groups and contexts, and how varied are the analytic and disciplinary approaches that can be adopted in exploring the overall theme. By reading all the chapters in the volume, readers will also begin to recognise whence the undergirding themes and issues that are highlighted in editorial introductory material and in the final chapter emerge.

We encourage all readers to read the papers from and about professions and disciplinary perspectives that are not most obviously relevant. In the authors' experience, this is probably how most intellectual satisfaction and fun is to be derived! We have often found that it is by approaching this topic tangentially, from a sideways rather than direct perspective, that the most interesting issues are rendered visible. Thus, reading about values in sport or planning may prove to be more stimulating for health and other caring professionals than reading the very substantial number of papers relating directly to those professions, challenging assumptions in a way that professional insiders cannot.

Some readers will simply want to start by reading about professions, topics or disciplinary approaches that are of particular interest to them. They will not lose out by doing this as each chapter is self-contained in itself.

All readers are advised to familiarise themselves with the concepts contained within the introductory chapters about values and professions which follow this. They are also encouraged to read the editorials that pertain to the parts of the book they are reading to ensure that they pick up wider issues and themes. It is hoped that the bibliography at the end of this volume will be of substantial help to any users who wish to pursue the relationships between professions and values further.

The background: how this book came to be

This volume is the result of collaborative research based round a group of ten academic researchers (many with a practice and training background) who have met together regularly to share papers and ideas over a period of three years from 2000 at Cardiff University. In terms of professional practice, we are all researchers, educators and trainers helping to develop practitioners, mainly for the public services and with a bias towards healthcare and the caring professions. We represent three different universities – Cardiff, Swansea and Birmingham. In terms of non-academic professional backgrounds, we are, or have been, three nurses, one planner, two clergy and two healthcare managers. With reference to the academic disciplines represented in the group we are thoroughly interdisciplinary and hybrid with interests in empirical research, sociology, philosophy, planning theory, nursing studies and practical theology, to name but a few of the more obvious interests and perspectives represented.

In addition to the core group, we have been fortunate to have the input of engineers, doctors, lawyers, journalists, sports professionals, leisure services managers, ethicists and others. Some members of this wider group have contributed chapters to this volume. The core group and around twelve other people met to discuss the themes and draft papers for this volume at a symposium held under the auspices of the Nuffield Trust in the summer of 2002. We hope in the future to expand this constituency of people interested in values and professions to include more professional and disciplinary perspectives such as those of politicians, school teachers, architects and any others who might be interested in our work. We will also try to engage in more empirical research.

This book, then, represents the first fruits of an ongoing collaborative, interdisciplinary endeavour to better understand the relationship of values and professional practice, both conceptually and empirically.

What is in the book

This book is not an encyclopaedia or a textbook. It aims to present critical issues about the relationship of values and professions from a variety of different academic and practitioner perspectives. There are thematic connections and relationships between the various chapters, however, so they are grouped together in different parts. These connections have emerged from interdisciplinary discussions so each theme in itself highlights up an important area of consideration or research that needs to be considered when approaching the relationship between values and professional practice. Each part has a short editorial introduction which briefly outlines each chapter and draws out emergent themes and issues.

The first two chapters, on values and professions respectively, provide basic orientation on these topics and the way that they are used and explored in subsequent chapters. This allows some initial explicit clarity about concepts and practices that might otherwise remain embedded in later material. Readers might like to return to them in the face of conceptual confusion and vertigo encountered in the chapters that follow.

Part I Professions and values in historical context

Many of the issues concerning the place of values in professions today can be illuminated by considering historical aspects of their evolution. This perspective is addressed here by considering the rise of the artistic profession and by examining the recent history of the clerical profession. By using these worked historical examples, issues about identity and professional values are thrown into relief. This provides an interesting contrast with the more conventional, normative evolution of the larger, more often considered professions such as law, medicine and nursing.

Part II Value conflicts and professional identity

The three chapters in this part of the book turn squarely to professional life and values in the contemporary world. They begin to explore the many tensions that exist in trying to manage and reconcile personal and professional values in institutional contexts, by focusing on public sector professionals in healthcare management, leisure services and social work.

Part III Values embodied in codes of practice

One popular way of embedding and identifying values in professional practice has been to codify them in written documents. In this part of the book, the virtue of codifying values is assayed and the uses and implications of the application of these codes – to guide, inspire, regulate and punish – are explored. The two chapters here consider two very different professional contexts and codes, those of nursing (a caring profession mostly in the public sector) and engineering (an environmentally related profession which relates often to the private sector). Some interesting commonalities and contrasts can thus be observed.

Part IV Values in education and training

Perhaps one of the main reasons for articulating professional values is to try to influence and socialise occupational recruits. The chapters in this part examine the educational values and practices associated with two further contrasting professional groups, law and planning. Disturbing questions are raised here about formal and informal socialisation into articulated and unarticulated values in professional training.

Part V Values in research

Nearly all contemporary professions see themselves as evidence based and research aware. Effective, reflective practitioners are bidden to undertake research. But how is this influenced by personal and professional values, and what values support and are implicated in the process and outcomes of research? The two chapters in this part open up the nature of researching values and the values of research by reflecting on the experiences of a particular occupational group – nurses – and upon the experience of individual researchers themselves.

In a concluding chapter, we assess what has been revealed by the book as a whole. We try to draw some conclusions, and raise conceptual and practical questions for further empirical and theoretical work. We also point directions for further reflection and research for individual professionals in different contexts, for different professional groups, and for interested bystanders. Some suggestions will be made about the implications for practical education and training of professionals of the findings of the book.

Bibliography

Finally, there is a bibliography which provides a succinct but reasonably comprehensive range of further reading on the issues and topics raised throughout the book.

CHAPTER 1

Understanding values*

Stephen Pattison

Introduction

The language of values is ubiquitous in contemporary society. Everyone is deemed to have values, and to have a competent view on them. *Prima facie*, the possession of values is held to be a good thing. Value-driven organisations are thought to be admirable because of their clear convictions. Individuals who have a set of articulated values are often lauded over against others who are muddled or inarticulate about theirs. Politicians who talk up values are in vogue – so long as their lives are not lived in too flagrantly a contradictory manner to the values they commend. But what are values, and why do they command such uniform interest and respect at the present time?

I want here to problematise the notions of value and values and the uses to which these concepts are put. My working hypothesis is that the concept 'values' is one of those portmanteau concepts which chases after meaning, like 'community'. It derives its popularity and legitimacy from the fact that it is an apparently simple, universally accessible concept which has a simple unexceptional primary meaning (a value is something which people value) which conceals a large number of secondary meanings and understandings. This enables people to find in it many nuances of meaning and to use it in many different ways and contexts. The notions of value and values can easily slip, chameleon-like, between users and utterances, delighting all and offending none because most people do not take the trouble to think about what they actually mean in their own lives or those of others.

---

*This is a revised and expanded version of Pattison S (1998) Questioning values. *Health Care Analysis*. **6**: 341–51. It is reproduced here with the permission of the publishers, John Wiley and Sons.

Definitions of values

Having started with meanings, it is perhaps appropriate to start with the issue of definitions and then to look at synonyms for values.

The primary definition of the noun 'value' in the 1971 edition of the *Oxford English Dictionary* is firmly economic. The value of something is 'that amount of some commodity, medium of exchange, etc., which is considered to be equivalent of something else; a fair or adequate equivalent or return'. The verb 'to value' means 'to estimate or appraise as being worth a specified sum or amount'.

These definitions immediately prompt some observations:

1 The concept of value emerges basically from the world of economic exchange, or the market. Perhaps this is why it has come to prominence over the last 20 years.

2 The 1971 edition of the *Oxford English Dictionary* does not note the use of value to connote a moral context, though it does note the use of the term to evaluate persons and their merits. This suggests that the current dominant use of values in an essentially moral context is a relatively recent phenomenon. It would be interesting to know why this usage has come to prominence in this way over the last couple of decades. (It should also be noted, *en passant*, that while the use of 'values' to denote aspects of moral and social significance and behaviour is often dominant in contemporary usage, all values are not moral values. Thus there are aesthetic, theological and other kinds of values that play an influential part in the lives and behaviours of individuals and groups [Budd 1996]. However, it is basically the moral and social notions of values that are most in need of interrogation here.)

3 The notion of value or valuing something is relative in its very essence (Mackie 1977: 5ff). The value or estimate of something is not something fixed and objective, but transitory. Essentially, value is in the eye of the beholder, valuer or evaluator. At the core of the apparent concreteness of the notion of 'values', relativity is built in. Value and values are, then, not Platonic ideas or innate concrete realities, but rather transient and thoroughly embedded in a fluid process of change. Even those philosophers who want to assert some kind of independent objectivity for values have to concede that their development has elements of change and emergence in them (Grice 2001). It is the inner relativity obscured behind the apparent concreteness and static nature of the noun 'value' that provides the notions of value and values with much of their conceptual slipperiness. The concepts are, so to speak, thoroughly post-modern. They appear to refer to some kind of tangible external reality. However, this is illusory and they are thoroughly non-realist and at best only partially referential. Gold is only valuable to those who value gold – and

those who value gold may do so for many different reasons. The metal, being itself inanimate and an object, does not require people to value it.

4   Talk of gold brings me to thoughts of 'standards' and the way in which this particular metal is taken by many to underwrite and guarantee the economic order. A similar intrinsic and unconscious positive valuation of the concept of 'value' as worthwhile in itself seems to perform an analogous purpose within the social and moral order. If we have values then all will be well. However, as is well known, all that glitters is not gold. Gold cannot perform many important functions, for example it is not a good material for cooking with. The notion that somehow values in and of themselves will form a foundation for life and the social order is a (perhaps necessary) illusion. While illusions and faith systems may indeed be necessary for individual and social functioning, the belief in values must be recognised as just such a faith system. The reification of values to the status of pre-existent, indispensable entities is an act of human creation – or, indeed, valuation.

Synonyms for values

The foregoing preliminary observations have highlighted the relativity and conceptual slipperiness of the notions of value and values outside the economic realm. They provide a valuable framing perspective on some of the synonyms and alternative words that often seem to be used alongside or instead of the words themselves. It will be noted that some of these synonyms, substitutes and associated words are far from having the positive, desirable and solid resonances that so often surround the concept of 'values' itself.

Preferences, choices and desires

This group of words comes from the economic domain where it is thought that what people prefer, desire or choose is what they value or confer worth upon. What is preferred, desired or chosen is what people are prepared to pay for and so value. To find out what people value, one must look for what they choose and express a desire for, or more concretely, what they will pay for. It is this set of meanings that often dominates in discussion of values in the public policy arena (Aaron *et al*. 1994).

Attitudes and beliefs

From the psychological domain come the notions of attitude and belief. From this perspective, what people are attitudinally predisposed towards, or believe in, whether they articulate it or not, is what they value. Attitudes and beliefs, and the values that they uphold or sustain, can be discerned by watching people's behaviours, e.g. voting for a particular party in an election, as well as by asking them what they believe in or are well-disposed towards.

Norms, assumptions, expectations, judgements and prejudices

Social norms, assumptions, expectations, judgements and prejudices are the province of sociology. They are what holds people together in groups so that society is coherent and individual behaviour is to some extent predictable and conformist. Embedded in social norms, assumptions, judgements and prejudices are shared views of what is good and bad, desirable and undesirable. Interestingly, values in common parlance are often presented as desirable while assumptions are questionable! I have values – you have assumptions and prejudices. The person with values may be thought of as moral, while the person with assumptions may be perceived to be unthinking or uncritical. This is just one instance of the phenomenon of value and values being differently evaluated and perceived according to the vocabulary used.

Standards, visions and goals

The world of management and manufacturing provides the concepts of standards, visions and goals that relate closely to those of value and values. Standards are norms of what is expected and required – they make clear what sufficient value will be from the perspective of the person who creates them. Visions provide ideal standards and points of reference to which the vision creators aspire – they point to the value that the vision maker wants to create (Pattison 1997: 62ff). Between visions and standards lie more proximate goals, or specific values targets which must be reached. Again, goals point to what is worthwhile and valuable.

Morals, principles and commitments

From the domain of ethics and morality come words like morals, principles and commitment. Morals are precepts and habits that are oriented towards attaining what is good and desirable, i.e. what is valued. Principles embody values and are designed to ensure that certain values are realised. Commitments can be intellectual and/or emotional, conscious and unconscious, theoretical or enacted ('I belong to the Conservative Party but I don't do anything for them'). They are the form of active consent to and the prosecution of values so that values are potentially concretised in some way. If one can find out what a person or group's principles and commitments are, then one has gone a good way towards identifying their values. Principles and commitments, unlike norms and prejudices, often have a halo of virtue attached to them though in fact these words are in many ways synonymous; this can be seen by substituting one set of words for the others. The real difference and distinction, which does of course exist between words, lies in matters of nuance, connotation and context surrounding particular terms and their usage in specific contexts. Thus prejudice may be regarded as more or less automatically 'blind', while commitment may implicitly be nuanced with notions of enlightenment.

There are many other terms that act as synonyms or are closely associated with values. Ideas, virtues and goods are further examples of terms that act much like values within the world of moral philosophy.

Virtue is a particularly important concept in the present context. Virtues are the habits and attitudes embedded in the characters of individuals that embody the positive ends and values towards which they aspire (Crisp and Slote 1997; Pence 1991). It is by persons adopting and habitually conforming to certain values in the interest of pursuing certain visions or ends that they become habitual virtuous performers. This is a primary means whereby values and value choices become enacted and incarnated in everyday life and professional practice.

Thus, a nurse who believes in respecting all people (valued end or vision) may think communication with patients to be a vital tool to making this a reality in everyday practice (valued means). They may train themselves habitually to listen to people very carefully. If they succeed in listening they become habitually and unselfconsciously a good communicator. They thus become a virtuous communicative person within the particular aspiration of developing the positive virtue of being able to listen. This within the teleology of trying to develop and maintain respect for all.

Training in virtues allows certain values, habits and attitudes to become second nature, part of the person's essential character (Hauerwas 1981). Virtuous, value-enacting behaviour is more than a matter of following rules. Thus values become incarnated as personal and professional virtues within particular individual characters. If a person is habitually committed to negative or harmful values and enacts these from their character, they can be said to demonstrate vices (bad habits) rather than virtues (Schimmel 1997). Whether a person is deemed to be of virtuous or of vicious character, the point is that values are integrally linked to personal identity. In a sense, one cannot help being the embodiment of one's values.

Definitions of values

Enough has now been said to highlight the problematic nature of defining and understanding the meaning of value and values and to substantiate the assertion that these terms have a slippery, chameleon-like nature. This perspective is useful when approaching definitions of values such as the following:

- A value is 'something we hold dear' (Keep and McClenahan 2002: 197).
- A value is an affective disposition towards a person, object or idea.
- A value is something we recognise as good and worthwhile.
- A value is a personal belief or attitude about the truth, beauty or worth of any thought, object or behaviour.
- Values appear as attributes of things and events themselves rather than as an activity of the self or as the result of such activity of the self or as the result or such activity (Tschudin 1992: 24).

In the light of the discussion above about words, it will be recognised that many of these definitions of value and values are at best partial and often simply arbitrary and even misleading. In particular, they are heavily weighted towards what I have identified as the psychological domain and basically away from that of the sociological or economic domains. This is not necessarily very helpful in trying to gain a reasonably complete picture of what values might be in human life and language.

An interesting definition of values that appears in Tschudin's workbook on identifying and working with values comes from the author herself. It is much less limited and mysterious, while remaining intriguing, than any of those quoted above:

- Values are closely related to meaning – the meaning of life. The inner meaning of an action, an experience or an attitude gives us our values (Tschudin 1992: 2).

This definition preserves the perception that values are created by human beings and are, therefore, situated within the realm of human meanings. At the same time, it maintains a sense of the relative incomprehensibility and uncircumscribable nature of values with the notion of inner meanings. As creatures who live and breathe meanings, it is very difficult for us to stand outside them and survey them dispassionately, least of all when they concern the fundamental way in which we perceive and operate in the world. Just as we breathe air and cannot see or describe it in any very nuanced way, we mostly breathe values and meanings, assuming them rather than interrogating their nature.

What is missing explicitly in Tschudin's definition is the degree to which individuals commit themselves emotionally to values, though it can be argued that individuals are necessarily very committed to inner meanings. People certainly suffer much emotional pain when values and fundamental meanings are threatened, lost, or disparaged. A good *via negativa* procedure for discovering what an individual or group's basic values and meanings are is to notice or ask them what distresses them or makes them unhappy in their life and work. Here again we can note the close relationship between values and fundamental personal and professional identity.

The nature of values

The foregoing discussion reveals a wide diversity of understandings and definitions that surround the concepts of value and values. It might be concluded that these notions only retain the sway they possess because people fail to examine their meanings and usage. Thus people can talk past each other while using the same words. It is not surprising, then, given fundamental conceptual confusion, that there is often fundamental confusion about values in practice. More analysis needs to be undertaken to create typologies of the meaning and nature of value and values. This is not the place, however, to outline such a typology or to start trying to develop a detailed understanding of the qualities and natures of particular kinds of values.

Nevertheless, one basic comment on the distinction between different kinds and usages of the term 'value' can usefully be made here. This is the distinction between what might be called 'normal' values and what might be designated 'aspirational' values. Both kinds of values are highly valued but they behave in rather different ways.

'Normal' values

'Normal' values are close to the sociological notion of norms, rules, habits, expectations and assumptions. They are the bricks and mortar of the everyday social world, comprising the basis of the worldview upon which human affairs are conducted. As such, they are mostly unexceptionable and unnoticed, do not require active commitment (though they may require active decommitment if a person wishes to escape from or challenge them) and appear to be so much a part of reality that one could not do without them. It would be wrong to think, however, that they do not have effects upon human behaviour and that they do not have an affective aspect, however humdrum they may be.

These 'normal' values, often associated with social conformity and leading a 'respectable' life, can arouse enormous passion and interest if they are challenged. When 'normal' values of bringing up children, dealing with strangers, conducting business, etc. are challenged or problematised, then people can become very upset, defensive, hurt and angry. These values go to the centre of personal and social identity in particular contexts. They may be deeply, if not consciously and passionately, held. Thus, exiles in alien cultures may suddenly discover that they are 'British' or 'Indian', becoming very conscious of threats to values and identity when these things are challenged in a way that they would not be if they had stayed in their culture of origin.

'Normal' values function much like some domestic object such as a shoe scraper. Mostly they are ignored and unused, but they are missed, with irritation, if found to be absent or stolen when it is confidently expected that they will be there. Moreover, those who are unaware of their presence may fall over them with quite damaging results. Anyone who has ever fallen over an unexpected shoe scraper will know exactly how much hurt and passion can be aroused by this!

Curiously, when politicians and others hark back to a past when traditional values were thought to have been present and talk of the need for fundamental, solid 'normal' values, e.g. the desire to support oneself by working, they bear witness to the endangered, fragile, relative and problematic nature of these values. It is only when they are threatened in some way that people talk about them. Like religion, 'normal' values function best when everyone accepts them to the point that they are not worth mentioning. When they are being discussed anxiously and very consciously, they are probably under threat of some kind.

'Aspirational' values

'Aspirational' values are close to notions of ideas, goals and visions and are values that are sought rather than assumed. They provide a yet-to-be-realised direction for life and society. They are likely to be quite conscious and people will probably have an overt emotional investment in them if they espouse them at all. Those who do not espouse them may have an emotional aversion to them that negatively images the positive investment of their proponents. 'Aspirational' values are likely to have the qualities of being freely chosen by individuals and groups from amongst alternatives and they are often overtly prized and proclaimed, as well as being consciously implemented in life and practice (Tschudin 1992: 27).

It is difficult to imagine a world without both 'normal' and 'aspirational' values as people value both stability and change, homogeneity and distinctiveness. Both kinds of values engage people's interest and emotions, but not in the same ways and circumstances. Clearly, it is possible for these different kinds of values to clash in very direct and painful ways. However, it would probably be a mistake to try to exalt one kind of value above the other. So, for example, it makes no real sense to disparage the conservative, assumed nature of latent 'normal' values just because they are not controversial or requiring direct assent in favour of 'aspirational' values that require conscious assent and overt ongoing expression and commitment. Both are needed, in their several ways.

It is worth noting in passing that often those who appeal to what appear to be 'normative' values that purport to represent past and tradition are in fact laying out a vision of 'aspirational' values that are designed to change the present and shape the future. This sleight of thought is readily apparent in political discourse. It forms a particularly important feature of the 'communitarian' critique of society and social institutions (Etzioni 1995a).

Some further features of values and their usage

If we could become clearer about what we mean by value and values, and also about the kinds and natures of values that are around, then our thinking and communications about these indispensable components of human life would be greatly facilitated. However, this would still leave a vast terrain of issues to explore further. Here are just some of the issues and tensions that I continue to ponder.

Values as a mixture of undifferentiated elements

It seems to me that to have any meaningful significance at all, values must attract a mixture of attitudes, beliefs, cognitions, affections and behaviours. Without any of these elements, values lose some of their reality and importance. However, it is not at all clear what proportions of these elements need to be present for a value to be said to have significance.

The origins and acquisition of values

Depending on one's view of what values are, it is possible to speculate on where they come from and how they are generated and reproduced. Andrew Wall, one of the authors contributing to this volume, suggests that many socially and morally significant values can be seen as being derived from three main sources. Some are *absorbed* from family and early socialisation. Others are *assimilated* from cultural norms of education, work and play. Finally some values are *acquired* from professional and legal codes and practices and conditions of work. He suggests that, correlatively, the need to reveal these values may vary accordingly from those which are felt to be personal, and to a degree, private, to those, which being attached to a particular working environment, are explicit but not necessarily well grounded or long-lasting within the self.

Anti-values?

Having said that values elicit a measure of commitment, whether active or passive (intellectual, affective, attitudinal, etc.), can there be such things as anti-values along the lines of antimatter in terms of physics or debt in terms of the market? Can things to which people are not committed or to which they are antagonistic be described as anti-values? If so, what effects do these disvalued things have on the social and moral world?

'Ropes' of values

It seems likely that most values do not exist in isolation, but form 'ropes' or perhaps 'constellations' within both individuals and social groups (Malby and Pattison 1999). At any one moment in time, certain values may be uppermost while others may be wholly or partially subordinated, just as constellations change in the night sky as the months go on. As far as I can see, we know little of how values are constellated, which adhere to which, for what reasons, and in what ways. We know even less about how and why they change in relative prominence in the lives of societies and individuals. Perhaps the sociologists can help here with their studies of social norms.

Conscious/unconscious, articulate/inarticulate values

Mostly people talk about values as if they have direct knowledge and access to them. However, often people's behaviour is at odds with their overt beliefs and convictions: organisations, too, often espouse values on paper (vision statements, missions, etc.) which are not enacted in practice. The questions here are: What relation do expressed and unexpressed values bear to each other? Are implicit enacted values as, or more, significant than explicit un-enacted values? What is the relationship of 'official' articulated values to unofficial values (e.g. healthcare facilities may claim to value their users and seek to do them good while actually being run for the convenience of the staff)? How can we find out what our real, i.e. operational and enacted, values are? Here again, there seems to be a deficiency of clarity and knowledge.

Changing values

It seems self-evident that many individuals and groups change their values over time. Also, they may often change their attitudes and relationships to values that remain basically constant over time. Perhaps in one day, talking or being with different people or groups, an individual might express and reprioritise their espoused values many times, obeying the rules of group norming and of explanation to an audience. It seems probable that people are likely to be engaged in a constant process of relative commitment and de-commitment to their values. Here again, we know little of what goes on and its significance for individuals and wider social groups.

Contradictory values

One of the interesting things about life is that one often encounters people who seem to be able to hold values that are on the face of it completely contradictory. So, for example, some right-wing Christians espouse the absolute value of life while advocating the death penalty for murderers. We appear to know little of how this apparent fundamental value clash is integrated in the individual given that they do not seem to suffer from any sense of cognitive dissonance as such.

The effect of values

Values as social norms have the effect of producing social consensus and regulation, while values as aspirational ideals provide a basic kind of direction. Over and above this, it is very difficult to say what values do and whether people who lack articulate or deeply held values, e.g. sociopaths, are deeply disadvantaged by this. What are the actual effects of values on individuals and groups?

The negative effects of values

It is sometimes assumed that values are a good thing in and of themselves and that they must, therefore, tend to have a beneficial effect upon those who hold them. It may even be assumed that the more tenaciously and firmly values are held, the more beneficent their effects will be. This is certainly not the case. Adolf Hitler had very strongly held values that he prized, but their effects on others were disastrous. Values are not unequivocally beneficent and good just by virtue of being values, nor are their effects necessarily positive, especially if they are placed in a properly relativistic perspective. Monolithic clarity about values can lead to the exclusion of important concerns, individuals and groups which can be very harmful, for example in public service which needs to be open to different cultures, values and interests (Pattison 1997, ch. 5). Rob Paton (1997) has demonstrated the ambiguous effects of strong values on voluntary organisations.

Values and stories

It seems to me that asking people directly what their values are is unlikely to elicit much knowledge about what values are operational in their lives as it concentrates only upon the cognitive aspect of values. If, as Alasdair MacIntyre suggests, we are narrative creating creatures and it is by this means that we manufacture and discover meaning in life, then it seems to me that it is worth considering stories and narratives as sources for discovering the values that people actually live by rather than those that they theoretically espouse (MacIntyre 1981: 201). Operant values worth studying are likely to be embedded in stories and practices rather than principles perhaps (Malby and Pattison 1999).

The social location of values

All values come from somewhere, are created by someone, and are espoused by particular groups and individuals. While there may be what passes for universal agreement on some values, such as the importance of life, it should be remembered that all values belong to some group or another and that it may be that another group's values may be ignored or ridiculed as a result. Values participate in power and influence struggle between groups. They do not stand above the social fray as an unequivocal court of certainty and appeal. The implication of this is that we need to become much more critical and conscious of where values come from, how they are formulated and used, and whose interests they serve.

The cost of values

To return to the economic market domain, whence value's primary use and meaning came, it should not be controversial to point out that valuing some things over others has a cost. Some things become sought after and desirable while others are denigrated and discarded. This may have a real cost to individuals and groups. It certainly seems to be the case that if workers in public service are caught with the wrong values, they feel uncomfortable and fundamentally rejected. In this sense, they pay the cost of the introduction of new values. It is probably always worth asking the question: Who pays the cost for my/our values?

Conclusion

The whole subject of values is surrounded by partiality, ignorance, confusion and ambiguity from the conceptual level down to that of everyday practice. Some of these problems have been exposed in a preliminary way here. A great deal more, and more detailed, work at conceptual and practical levels needs to be undertaken before we can really start to talk intelligibly and in a non-confusing way about value and values. One thing is clear: we will never completely escape from the relativity and conceptual slipperiness that inheres in the very nature of valuing some things over others. Values are created and interpreted in an ongoing dynamic process, not revealed. In the short term, however, this knowledge will not convince politicians, professionals and professions that values may not be in and of themselves a wholly desirable thing.

CHAPTER 2

Understanding professions and professionals in the context of values

Roisin Pill, Paul Wainwright, Michael McNamee and Stephen Pattison

Introduction

Who exactly are the 'professionals'? What do we understand by terms such as profession, professional, professionalisation and professionalism?

Like the concepts 'value' and 'values', terms like profession, professional and professionalism can be variously understood. Here, then, is another slippery set of concepts with a penumbra of associations and meanings. It is important to know something of the complexity of meaning and understanding surrounding professions to be able to orient oneself clearly within the debate about values and their place in occupational life today.

In this chapter we first look more closely at these words, their multiple meanings, how they are defined, and the way they are used in everyday life. Then we present, briefly, two very different approaches to understanding the professions and professional activity. One is grounded in social science. It highlights organisational and structural aspects of understanding the social evolution and functioning of professions as institutions. The other is based in philosophy. It highlights the moral significance of professions and the goods that they might seek, and particularly the character of individual professionals as virtuous agents.

The accounts of these two approaches are not comprehensive, nor can they necessarily be synthesised into a unified account of professions and professionalism. They are presented here to show how different disciplinary traditions have tackled concepts of professions and professionalism. They each provide some ideas and insights which help provide orientation to the complex issues surrounding the nature of professions and professionalism today.

Profession, professionals and professionalism: some problems with language

In everyday conversation the terms 'profession', 'professional' and 'professionally' are widely used. However, the examples given below show that the underlying meaning may be interpreted in very different ways by listeners, depending on the context and previous experiences or expectations they hold. For example:

'She did a professional job'
The task was well executed and competently done.

'Speaking professionally'
This speaker is making a claim to attention (possibly also respect and deference) by virtue of their particular expertise and their higher educational qualifications. Maybe this person is trying to make me feel inferior or make themselves more superior.

'He behaved very professionally'
He was courteous, objective, unemotional; he went out of his way to help me; I am confident that he will not betray my trust or confidences.

'I always do a professional job'
I deserve more status/money; my job is important, worthwhile, etc.

These brief examples reveal some of the possible range of meanings that terms like 'professional' can have in everyday parlance. The picture gets more complicated.

Further ambiguities arise in the use of words like these because a word is being made to do two or more different jobs if it carries with it a great deal of 'baggage' by way of secondary or unintended meanings. The term 'profession' can be used as a very defined, narrow quasi-scientific concept. Thus a social scientist may want to use it as a neutral, descriptive term for one of the several forms of occupational organisation to be found in society. But as used in ordinary everyday discourse, it can suggest instead a morally desirable kind of work. Sociologist Howard Becker argues:

> Instead of resembling the biologist's conception of a mammal, it [profession] more nearly resembles the philosopher's or theologian's conception of a good man. It is a term of invidious comparison and moral evaluation; in applying it to a particular occupation people mean to say that the occupation is morally praiseworthy, just as in refusing to apply it to another occupation they mean to say that it is not morally worthy of the honour.
>
> (Becker 1970a: 90)

Some occupations describe themselves as professions. Other occupations might like to designate themselves thus, but find that no one else takes their claim seriously. Lay people habitually use the term to refer to certain kinds of work but not others, albeit that the tasks undertaken may be no less complex and the rewards no less great.

Because of the moral superiority that may be implicitly ascribed to occupations that have this label attached to them, many work groups seek the title 'profession'. This kind of moral loading of the term often distorts attempts at refining definitions to be more objective and specific.

Before going on to look further at the meanings of profession and its cognates, you might care to pause and reflect on your own use of terms such as the noun 'profession', the noun and adjective 'professional' and the adverb 'professionally'. How do you use them and for what purpose? What do you mean when you use words like these? Would you apply these words to yourself and your colleagues? In what contexts? And if you would not do so, *why* would you not do so?

Some definitions

A dictionary definition is a crystallisation of many years of usage, shaped by the users of the language. The *Shorter Oxford English Dictionary* (1983) provides two main definitions of 'profession' which reflect some of the ambiguities already noted above. One is quite narrow and specific in focus. The other is much broader, effectively equating profession with occupation:

1   the occupation which one professes to be skilled in and to follow, a vocation in which a professed knowledge of some department of learning is used in the application to the affairs of others, or in the practice of an art founded upon it – applied especially to the three learned professions of divinity, law and medicine; also to the military profession
2   any calling or occupation by which a person habitually earns his living.

The fact that the word 'profession' can be used both specifically and more generally highlights the potential complexity of the concept and the need to examine more closely the context in which it is being used to be clear about its meanings.

The first, narrower definition implies the following:

● claims to particular expertise and skill
● a sense of calling (as opposed to simply working for money)
● the need for learning or grasp of theoretical knowledge
● service to others
● restriction to certain categories of occupation only – this may also imply enhanced social status.

The same dictionary defines 'professionals' thus: 'persons engaged in one of the learned or skilled professions, or in a calling considered socially superior to a trade or handicraft'.

There are very clear similarities here with the narrower definition of profession cited above. These include:

- more education or training
- special expertise
- readiness to serve others altruistically
- the approbation and respect of fellow citizens.

By contrast, the second definition of profession cited effectively makes no distinction between profession and occupation. It emphasises the fact that an individual is remunerated for the service provided. The distinction is drawn between those who earn their living by providing a specific service and those who are unpaid volunteers or amateurs. There is also, of course, a possible tension between the two definitions: the professional as the beneficent dispenser of expertise versus the professional as dependent on fees from others to survive.

The *Shorter Oxford English Dictionary* goes on to define 'professionalism' as 'professional quality, character, method or conduct'. Thus Irvine (1997: 1540), discussing the training of doctors, declares that, 'The everyday behaviour of clinical teachers is the living demonstration of their expertise, ethics and commitment: their professionalism'. Here, not only are claims being made about the technical competence, moral authority, dedication and possible altruism of the clinical teacher. A link is explicitly being made between observed behaviour and the values held by the individual.

Understanding the meaning of professions as social symbols

The question 'what is a profession?' is an old one (Becker 1970a: 87). No absolute consensus has been reached as to what this term specifies. Becker proposed that those studying the professions should treat the notion as a folk concept, a part of the apparatus of the society being studied. They should concentrate on noting how the term is used and what *symbolic* part it plays in the operation of that society.

In this type of social symbolic analysis, the focus is on the conventional social beliefs and assumptions of what the characteristics of a profession *ought* to be. Becker argues that it is this model on which people draw, whether they are members of recognised professions themselves or of aspiring occupational groups, clients or part of the general public.

> The symbol of the ideal profession consists of a set of ideas about the kind of work done by a real profession, its relations with

members of other professions, the internal relations of its own members, its relations with clients and the general public, the character of its own members' motivations, and the kind of recruitment and training necessary for its perpetuation.

(Becker 1970a: 93).

Key to this socio-symbolic understanding of professions are the following beliefs:

- monopoly of some esoteric and difficult body of knowledge considered necessary for the continuing functioning of society
- the recruitment and lengthy training of carefully selected individuals with the appropriate personal qualities to apply their expertise wisely
- selection, education and regulation procedures being carried out by members of the profession and therefore outside lay control
- the altruistic motivation of members and the strict enforcement of a code of ethics emphasising devotion to service and the good of the client
- the client's complete trust in the integrity and competence of the professional
- the image of the profession and the professional as occupying an esteemed position in society.

No occupational group precisely corresponds to this ideal symbolic type of the profession. Insofar as Becker is correct, and this set of beliefs does inform and underpin people's views, expectations and judgements, there is potential for considerable dissonance between expectations and actual experience both for the professionals and those they encounter. Many of us in our lay capacity would, for example, be able to recognise dissonance between the aspiration to altruism and what sometimes seems to be the self-interested behaviour of some professions and professionals.

Professions and professionals: some sociological perspectives

It is not possible or desirable to give a full account of the many sociological writings that have been published on the nature and functioning of professions. A copious literature testifies to the perceived social importance of this topic in the eyes of numerous academics and commentators. Here, some of the main approaches are briefly outlined.

Professions as social institutions

Professions can be thought of as examples of social phenomena or institutions. (By institution here we do not mean simply a building or a particular organisation but, following the *Shorter Oxford English Dictionary*, a much broader sense of that word as 'an established law, custom, usage, practice, organisation or other element in the political or social life of a people'.)

Medicine is often used as an example to advance theories of the professions as institutions. It has been taken as the epitome of what 'profession' means and will be used to illustrate the theoretical approaches below (Friedson 1970). Even so 'there is no consensus about how medicine is to be understood or its social history or current situation explained' (Coburn and Willis 2000: 378).

Examination of what has been written about the professions in general and medicine in particular reveals the changing fashions in sociological approaches over the years.

Trait theories

This approach, popular in the mid-twentieth century, attempted to produce a neutral, objective definition that would distinguish the professions as one of the several forms of occupational organisation in society. All professions were deemed to possess certain common attributes or traits which identified them as professions. The traits often identified included: an esoteric specialist body of knowledge; a code of ethics; an altruistic orientation (Carr-Saunders and Wilson 1933; Greenwood 1957). It was also argued that professions moved through a sequence of the acquisition of particular traits as they developed (Wilensky 1964).

Trait theories were developed by comparison of common-sense notions of professions (derived from the generally recognised professions of medicine and law) with the assumed characteristics of other occupations. By including altruism as an essential attribute of professions, i.e. the professionals viewing themselves as working for the good of society, trait theorists implied that professions were morally praiseworthy in a way other occupations were not.

Theories about the relationship of the professional to clients and the wider society

For some analysts the key feature for understanding professions and professionals was the particular moral relationship of trust with their clients and wider society. This was compared with the morality of businessmen whose interest in profit was the underlying motive for a different kind of behaviour. Hence an 'implicit contract' between society and the professions, particularly the medical profession, was postulated whereby the latter were allowed autonomy in exchange for stringent self-regulation (Parsons 1951).

Generally, professionals were perceived as altruistic. The growth of the professions was regarded positively as contributing to the 'modern' society. However, as it became clear that the professions were often not as self-regulated or altruistic as had been claimed, writers became more critical. Professions were perceived as potentially exploitative monopolies, a 'conspiracy against the laity'. Critics like Ivan Illich (1976) even went so far as to suggest that professions like medicine were positively harmful, causing harm ('iatrogenic') and disabling those they ostensibly sought to help.

For the medical profession, a key figure in constructing this critique of altruism was Friedson (1970). He argued that the profession fundamentally acted in its own interest to preserve and confirm a position of dominance in society and the healthcare sector. It appealed to its service orientation and scientific expertise to legitimate its mandate and autonomy. Medical dominance meant that the profession controlled both the content of medical work and the clients, other healthcare professions, and the context within which healthcare was given, including healthcare policy.

Power theories

The subsequent debate resulted in alternative interpretations of the power of the medical profession (Coburn and Willis 2000) and also in empirical research studies. The focus shifted to how certain occupational groups obtained and maintained their power to define their sphere of expertise, to control practice, and to resist attempts to usurp their authority in different and changing social and economic contexts.

Medicine, for example, has long been at the apex of a whole range of health professions and occupations. It has gained the power to exclude, limit or subordinate its potential rivals. This 'system of health professions' (Abbott 1988) provides examples of aspirant professions such as hospital managers and the paramedical occupations, and of inter-occupational strife involving the renegotiation of boundaries between groups, e.g. doctors and nurses.

Similar issues of demarcation concerning the professional domain can be observed in other professional fields. In law there have been boundary disputes among barristers, solicitors and legal executives. In education, too, there have been arguments about the relative positions and responsibilities of teachers and classroom assistants. In these cases, as in medicine, there have been attempts to barricade or break down professional domains and to preserve or destroy perceived privileged or hierarchical relations.

Current debates

Interest has turned more recently to the possible decline of the professions and how this may be understood (Broadbent *et al.* 1997). For example, much has been written about the decline of medical dominance in Britain and North America and the rise of other occupational groups such as psychology and nursing. Some writers argue for a trend towards the proletarianism of medicine (McKinlay and Stoeckle 1988; Salmon 1994). Others argue that medicine has simply changed its form or nature (Elston 1991; Larkin 1993). It is, however, generally accepted that shifts in both the broader economic and political situation are bound to affect the profession of medicine and, of course, other professions and occupations as well.

Professions today: a new sociological approach

The American sociologist Brint (1994) has explored the question of the changing roles of the professions in advanced capitalist societies. He argues that professions and professionalism should be seen as historically evolving sociological forms. Brint's interest is in the 'professional middle class', people who earn at least a middling income from the application of a relatively complex body of knowledge. In the USA this group has grown dramatically in the last 30 years. Its members are increasingly visible in public life. Similar trends are apparent in other Western industrial societies.

Brint argues that:

> Modern professions are a product of the dynamic era of white-collar professionalisation encompassing roughly the century between 1860 and 1960. The period can be characterised as one in which a great many white-collar occupations – from engineers to social workers – sought 'collective mobility' through efforts to emulate the 'established professions' of medicine, law, theology and the professariat.

He goes on:

> The professions, alone among occupations, rely on higher education as a requisite for access to markets. This institutional fact has created conditions for a certain number of common powers and privileges, the most widespread of which has been autonomy in relation to how work has been conducted.
>
> (Brint 1994: 5–6)

Because of historical changes since about 1960, the idea of professionals as agents of formal knowledge has largely superceded the idea of professionals as 'trustees' of socially important knowledge. During the dynamic age of expansion professionalism as an ideology had both a technical and a moral aspect. Technically, it promised competent performance of skilled work involving the application of broad and complex knowledge, the acquisition of which required formal academic study. Morally, it promised to be guided by an appreciation of the important social ends it served. In demanding high levels of self-governance, professionals claimed not only that others were not *technically* equipped to judge them but also that they could not be *trusted* to judge them (Brint 1994: 7).

Because of its inclusive nature, this set of beliefs proved helpful to the emerging white-collar professions:

> Occupations like school teaching and social work with dubious technical capacities could nevertheless claim a kind of moral superiority and look forward to further technical achievements as an important aspiration. Others like engineering with a more secure technical base often found it convenient to identify themselves as serving larger social purposes.
>
> (Brint 1994: 7)

Brint suggests that there was always a rival idea of professions. Here the emphasis was on intellectual training in the service of purposes determined by organisational authorities or market forces. This rival idea has now become dominant. Over the last three decades, the idea of professions has become increasingly disconnected from functions central to public welfare. It is now more exclusively connected to the idea of 'expert knowledge'. Where professionals see themselves primarily as 'experts' or 'specialists', the notion of social contribution has little intrinsic meaning. It is assumed that it can be measured by the market value of specialised skills. This is associated to closer links between the major professions and business and the weakening of barriers to the pursuit of profit in openly competitive markets. What remains of social trustee professionalism has become associated almost exclusively with the public and non-profit sectors.

This shift has caused a split in the ever increasing number of those who could/might be categorised as 'professional'. There is now:

- a stratum of upper-level experts definable by the combination of marketable skills and location in resource-rich organisations
- a stratum of lower-level experts definable by the combination of less marketable skills and location in resource-poor organisations.

Brint argues these connections of professionals to markets and organisations have become as important as the similarities that remain among them, namely, being a 'credentialled body of producers of "expert services" organised around a body of formal knowledge and claiming authority on that basis' (Brint 1994: 205). The connections and their implications will need more theoretical and empirical analysis if we are to reach a better understanding of modern professions, professionals and their values.

Professionals and their practice: a philosophical perspective

The social science commentaries and critiques discussed above have tended towards understanding professional organisational structures and issues such as power, dominance, socio-historical context and evolution. In the philosophical arena, by contrast, there has been a tendency to focus on the *nature* and *purpose* of contemporary professional activity, goods and necessary virtues. Professional behaviour and its associated values have been emphasised here, along with understanding of the virtues needed by individual practitioners.

Moral philosopher Alasdair MacIntyre makes a seminal contribution to the current debate about professional behaviour and values in his book *After Virtue* (1981). Here MacIntyre develops a contemporary account of the moral virtues, not primarily an account of the professions. While he uses professions such as medicine to illustrate his arguments, his account is focused on the defining *goods* of social activities, each of which are committed to a set of internal values. One of the most important concepts he developed in relation to the activities of professionals is the notion of 'professional practice'.

The definition of a practice

For MacIntyre (1981: 175), a practice is:

> any coherent and complex form of socially established co-operative human activity through which goods internal to that form of activity are realised in the course of trying to achieve those standards of excellence which are appropriate to, and partially definitive of, that form of activity, with the result that human powers to achieve excellence, and human conceptions of the ends and goods involved, are systematically extended.

He argues that 'the range of practices is wide: arts, sciences, games, politics in the Aristotelian sense, the making and sustaining of family life, all fall under the concept' (MacIntyre 1981: 175). This definition can include the traditionally constituted professions. Practices are defined by their purpose, their goals or ends, not by descriptions of tasks or skills. They are not static, but evolve constantly, informed by a critical sense of their traditions. Any meaningful account of a practice will take the form of a narrative, with a sense of both continuity and evolution.

MacIntyre specifically mentions medicine, education and sports among other social practices that can also be the site of professions and professionalism. (For examples of applications of these models, see Dunne [1993] on education; Morgan [1994] on sports; Solomon [1993] on business.)

MacIntyre's approach is strongly normative. For an activity to be characterised as a social practice, it must be co-operative, it must seek to achieve standards of excellence, and it must promote goods internal to the practice, such as health, knowledge, justice and so on.

There are further internal goods in the shape of the inherent rewards available to the practitioner who engages in distinctive practices. These include the satisfaction that comes with mastery of one's professional skills and success in achieving the goods and ends to which the practice is directed in society. But these, crucially, are dependent upon the presence, in the practitioner, of basic moral virtues:

> A virtue is an acquired human quality, the possession and exercise of which tends to enable us to achieve those goods which are internal to practices and the lack of which effectively prevents us from achieving any such goods.
>
> (MacIntyre 1981: 178)

The virtuous practitioner

According to MacIntyre, all virtuous practitioners in whatever profession must necessarily possess the generic virtues of honesty, courage and justice. If they do not, they cannot achieve the internal, intrinsic goods inherent in their particular practice. This is because without the generic virtues or qualities, they will not be able to preserve the space and character of the distinctive inherent goods of their particular practices from external forces.

Of course, successful practitioners may also be rewarded with goods external to the practice. These are the material rewards like money, power and prestige. They differ from internal goods intrinsic to practices in several important ways. For example, they are available in finite amounts. The more of these goods that accrue to one individual, mostly the less there is for others. Furthermore, external goods can be obtained in many ways – there is nothing about the salary of a doctor or a lawyer that is specific to that profession. Similar amounts of the same kind of 'stuff' can be obtained by people by very different occupational activity. For MacIntyre, competition for these goods that are external to particular practices is always potentially corrupting. To the extent that society is driven by such competition for external goods, the internal virtues are likely to be absent.

Practices versus institutions

A further important distinction is the difference between practices and institutions (MacIntyre 1981: 181ff). Practices cannot exist independently of institutions such as professional bodies and organisations. But institutions serve very different purposes and agendas to practices. Often, these are related precisely to goods external to practices.

For example, institutions are typically responsible for the distribution of external goods, the awarding of rank and status, and the scaling of monetary rewards. Institutions also determine, or at least agree, the extent of a practice, granting a licence to practitioners to control certain aspects of our lives. Examples are those of engineering, farming, law, midwifery, nursing and teaching. Relevant institutions here include, but are not restricted to, the National Farmers' Union, the Law Society, the Royal College of Nursing, and the General Teaching Council.

To the extent that professions are self-regulating, retaining control over entry, qualifications, licence to practise, professional discipline and so on, they function as institutions and control external goods. Because they represent the arena within which the distribution of external goods is controlled, and because they may have different goals and agendas, the institution is potentially corrupting of individual professional practice and its intrinsic goods. The internally related goods of practice-oriented professionals are a counter-weight to this potential corruption.

There is a real tension here in practice as well as theory. This can be seen in the modern phenomenon of whistle-blowing (Hunt 1995; Davis 1996). Whistle-blowers are often virtuous practitioners who attempt to act out of and to preserve the intrinsic goods of their professional practice at the expense of having to criticise an encroaching institution which may be seen to be attempting to pervert this practice because of a commitment to more external, extrinsic goods (e.g. meeting budgetary targets, following government policy, gaining more financial rewards for members of the profession generally).

To resist the encroachment of potentially corrupting external goods mediated through institutional pressures on practice, professionals, as adherents of particular practices, must try to exercise a virtuous influence over the activities of their relevant institutions. This influence should celebrate and preserve, for example, the courage of the nurse caring for the dying patient, the honesty of the solicitor who does not bury key evidence in mountainous caseloads, or the integrity of the teacher who seeks to develop the wholeness of students as rounded educated people rather than narrowly focused examination-taking machines. By behaving thus in relation to institutions, practitioners can help to ensure that professions as corporate bodies can themselves attain and maintain virtue, not just the individual practitioners within them.

To retain a vision of morally praiseworthy professional practice requires setting out clearly the values that sustain good practice and nurture intrinsic goods and the virtues they require. We can begin to see a model emerging that may help to explain the relationship between values and the professions.

Different kinds of values and conflicting values

There are some generic virtues/values that all professionals need to hold or aspire to for practices to flourish and for the internal goods and values inherent in them to be promoted. These include the basic moral virtues of courage, honesty and justice which are not role- or profession-specific. They are the foundation for any professional practice and represent part of the 'ethical probity' of the profession (Friedson 1970).

Other generic virtues/values which allow any practice to flourish might include commitment to working competently, to improvement, to openness, to scrutiny and to appraisal by peers and others. This in the context of the specific skills, interventions, roles and ends that make up the practice of the profession.

Alongside the internally related virtues and values that allow professional practices to flourish must be placed externally related generic values. These are 'goods external' – money, power, fame and the other material goods that come from success. Such external goods are powerful motivators and markers of success. They also represent recompense for what may be difficult and demanding work of great public value.

To the extent that the human beings at the heart of these practices and institutions are driven by what we might crudely refer to as 'good values' – the moral virtues, altruism, the internal goods and virtues that are intrinsic to practice and that are of shared benefit to society and so on – we can see how the professions could be seen to function in a healthy way in society. To the extent that competition for external goods, market forces and a libertarian survival of the fittest dominates, there is a basic threat to these 'good values'.

There is a potentially dangerous competition for external goods that may threaten the corruption of the virtues and goods internal to practices. Thus to understand some of the main value conflicts in professional theory and practice today, it is necessary to keep in mind the potential conflict between the internal goods espoused by the professionals in their practices and those external goods and pressures that are evident in institutions and their management, e.g. the drive for effectiveness and efficiency, market forces and success measured by performance indicators.

Unsurprisingly, much of the recent debate around professions revolves around perceived threats to their existence and functioning such as trends towards globalisation, a general increase in the power of corporations, a decline in the relative autonomy of the state and concomitant attacks on the welfare state. All these factors challenge the internal 'good' values and virtues that professionals may seek to espouse and promote.

This brief analysis of the relation of virtuous practitioners to externally driven, potentially less virtuous institutions such as professional and managerial bodies allows a particular perspective on contemporary professions and professionals. However, it should be noted that this analytic framework based on MacIntyre's is itself value-laden. It assumes a communitarian view of the world (Etzioni 1995b). Here the well-being and flourishing of communities relying on values of mutual solidarity and interdependence is privileged over the promotion of individual freedom, consumerism and liberty. This is a context in which, for example, individuals and professionals might trade commodities with each other in a direct consumer–supplier relationship. A different kind of philosopher, e.g. a libertarian who emphasised individual freedom and autonomy, could come up with a very different framework for understanding professional values and practice today.

Conclusion

In comparing these examples of the sociological and philosophical approaches, a striking difference lies in the nature of the questions posed and the type of analysis undertaken.

Sociologists have largely concentrated on 'the professions' as organisations and professionals as important groups in society. They have been concerned to understand and theorise about their evolution, structure and culture, and have attempted to account for change in professions as distinctive social groups. Sociological analysis emphasises the wider context in which organisations and individuals operate and the external economic and political pressures influencing them over time. Empirical work is used to test and generate theories and to identify the gaps between the idealised claims made by professional organisations and experiences of actual practice and behaviour found in observations and accounts provided by clients, the general public and by professionals themselves.

By contrast, the philosophical approach considered is more concerned with analysing 'the professional', i.e. the individual practising a particular expertise, and debating what attributes, values and virtues it would be desirable for such individuals to possess. This work is more theoretical and strongly normative. Professionals are of interest in this perspective because they are viewed as being situated in a moral ecology in which it is believed that they should demonstrate and defend morally significant activity which is of importance not just to the practitioner but also to society at large, e.g. the realisation of health, of justice, of education. The philosophical approach thus reflects theoretically upon the nature and attributes of the 'virtuous practitioner'.

When considering the interrelationship between the concepts of values and professions, the empirical emphasis versus the theoretical/normative focus of the two approaches becomes even more evident. Sociologists have been concerned to explore what values have been attributed to the group of occupations labelled professions by the rest of their society at a particular point in time and to understand the implications of such attributions. They have also been interested in how specific values are espoused by those in traditional professions seeking to maintain their position and those in other occupations seeking to improve theirs. In other words, sociologists have mostly documented the way that values are attributed and used in inter-occupational struggles for power and status in a given society by the members of that society. They have then sought to provide theories to explain these findings, particularly stressing the importance of a changing social context.

Philosophers are more likely to start by considering what moral virtues and values might be desired or required of someone doing an important job in our society given the need to promote certain overall ends of enabling corporate human flourishing. Rather than simply describing what is the case in the way of professional and occupational practice and trying to explain it, they have tried to present a wider ideal vision within which occupational values and virtues should be situated and even to prescribe what values and virtues should be manifested. The philosophical task is thus in the first instance to set a reasonable ideal before the rest of society.

Both sociologists and philosophers are well aware of the gap between ideal and reality. Both seek to explain it by reference to the context in which the professional is working, taking into account historical context, organisational constraints, etc. While philosophers may be more focused on individuals, the role of organisations and their effects on the possibilities for individual realisation of practice values are not ignored. Thus, there is a need for organisations or institutions to be involved in thinking about wider moral values, issues and tasks – a task which may be realised in the mechanisms, codes and mission statements whereby institutions like professional bodies and organisations articulate their own values, norms and standards of belief and behaviour.

The importance of considering both sociological and philosophical approaches selectively in the present context is that it makes clear that there are very different ways of understanding the complex, even contradictory, nature and values of professions and professionals. In practice, most of us, whether we are professionals or their clients, probably veer between holding views of what professions and professionals should be (a normative approach) and knowing something of what happens in reality (a descriptive approach). Often we conflate the two approaches in what might be called an uncritical 'common-sense approach' to professions and professionals, their behaviours and values.

The purpose of separating out these ways of analysing professionals and professions here has been to help readers to be more self-conscious of the assumptions that they might make about these matters, to reveal something of the range of ways of analysing them, and to provide a framework for understanding some of the tensions that can arise in theory and practice between ideal and reality, the individual practitioner and the institutional body. Together with the preliminary analysis of everyday language about the nature of professions and professionals using common definitions, this should have vindicated the initial assertion that here we are not only dealing with ambivalent slippery meanings, but also with very different ways of understanding the place and values of professions in social life.

This is not just a matter of bringing dizzying conceptual complexity into a discussion about professions and professionals for the sake of it. The different values and behaviours that might result from different ideals and realities can bring painful dilemmas for practitioners and professional bodies as they try to discern and live out their values in the morally complex, pluriform context of modern Western society.

PART I

Professions and values in historical context

Introduction

Much of the time many of us tend only to think of the professions that we know or belong to. We may assume that they have always been much the same in terms of values and practices as we find them today. We may have large paradigmatic professional groups in our minds such as law, medicine or nursing. Perhaps we may think, if we think about it at all, that they have always been more or less as they are.

The purpose of this book is to try to problematise assumptions about professions and values. Paradoxically, however, if this topic is engaged with head on, it may not always be easy to see what the main issues are. In particular, if people continue to think only of a narrow range of familiar groups in the context of the present, it can be very difficult to see the wood for the trees. If, however, a sideways look is taken, beyond the main professional groups and contemporary issues that come most immediately to mind, then some interesting questions and perceptions about professions and their relationships with values begin to emerge.

In this part of the book, readers are invited to challenge their assumptions about the origins, values and practices of professions by looking at and thinking about two fascinating historical accounts of professional change and development. The first example is that of the rise of artists aspiring to move from artisan status to gain influence and status as a professional group in affluent society in the eighteenth and nineteenth centuries. The second is the recent fate of clergy in British society, particularly their changing role and status as they lost their automatic significance amongst the ruling classes and have begun to de-professionalise and diversify in a number of ways.

In Chapter 3 'Professionalisation and aesthetic values', Andrew Edgar, a philosopher of art as well as an ethicist, charts the rise and discourse of artists as they sought to become full members of polite middle class society in the late eighteenth and nineteenth centuries so that they could sell their non-useful wares of fine art to a newly affluent group. The values at stake in this professional bid for significance were aesthetic values rather than the financial, altruistic or moral values that are associated with traditional helping professions today. Edgar recounts the ways in which artists like Sir Joshua Reynolds together with philosophers such as David Hume contributed to a discourse of good taste for an aspirant connoisseur class. Once this discourse, which built both on the notions of progress and development and also those of tradition and custom, was in place, both artists and their customers could participate in it as equals, being gentlemen of conversation and distinction. Newly gentrified artistic providers and their clients together could agree on each other's significance and acceptability and thus allow fruitful commercial and conversational exchanges to commence. The professionalisation of artists represents a well-orchestrated and planned bid for social and economic significance.

If eighteenth- and nineteenth-century artists form a good example of upward professional mobility and the formation of professional identity round a distinctive set of values shared by both providers and clients, clergy show a very different aspect of professional movement. Paul Ballard, a Baptist minister and theologian, reveals in Chapter 4 'The clergy: an interesting anomaly' the recent fate of one of the oldest learned professions in Western society. Two hundred years ago the higher clergy were amongst the most distinctive, affluent, influential and well-accepted occupational groups in society. Now, their place and fortunes are less secure and clear in contemporary secular culture with declining numbers of church members and less money to support the ministry of dedicated full-time workers. Since the last war numbers of full-time clergy have declined, methods of training them have diversified and now, arguably, they are in danger of not being regarded as a professional group at all, with many clergy (including some of the most able clergy) earning their livings in secular employment (Pattison 1989: 153ff). While they continue to maintain a clear base in theological values and a sense of vocation, the role and value of clergy as a professional group is now problematic. Ballard explores the reasons for these radical changes in the clerical role and professional identity and reveals some of the creative ways in which this group is responding to its marginalisation. He shows that the end of professional organisation as conventionally understood does not mean the end of distinctive values, nor of a valuable contribution to society.

What can be learned in general terms about professions and values that can be of value to those concerned with these matters from a non-artistic and non-clerical perspective? First, professions are in a constant state of flux. While occupational groups often present themselves as eternal and fixed by tradition, social utility and practice, they undergo a process of change; they wax and they wane. Secondly, this process is profoundly affected by changes in social values. Thus aestheticisation of the middle classes allows artists' status to increase while secularisation leads to the de-professionalisation of the clergy. Thirdly, the process of change and negotiation of social acceptability and status is directly related to the values of the profession or the occupational group itself. The legitimacy and significance of those values should not be underestimated in thinking about whether professions will rise, flourish or fall. Fourthly, and perhaps most significantly here, it is not just ethical or moral values that can be of huge importance in shaping the identity and fortunes of occupational groups in society. Theological, aesthetic and other non-moral values can have a crucial role in establishing the legitimacy and character of professions.

In more general terms, both of these chapters about the history of relatively marginal professions illustrate further issues that are of concern and interest to most, if not all, professional groups, whether historical or contemporary. The bid to become or remain a 'successful' or socially acceptable profession is strongly correlated with a range of issues that are directly related to values. Identity, power, status, legitimacy, the validity of different types of knowledge, the place of reason or faith, the capacity to make universally valid claims, the role and interpretation of tradition versus the need to change to keep up with changing social mores, the identification between individuals and professional bodies, the relationship between personal and organisational values and the nature of personal commitment or vocation, the nature of the 'virtuous' (i.e. trustworthy) practitioner, the essence of distinctively professional work which cannot be trusted to non-professionals, the place of money and extrinsic factors such as economics in shaping professional values and practices, all these are issues which confront not only clergy and artists but any occupational group that has been or aspires to the description 'profession'. These are themes emerging from a sideways glance at two historical examples, to which we shall return as the book progresses.

CHAPTER 3

Professionalisation and aesthetic values

Andrew Edgar

Introduction

The professional status of any occupation or trade is rarely, if ever, self-evident. It may be suggested that those occupations that have achieved the status of a profession do so, typically, only after a protracted process of negotiation. Debates within the occupation and between the occupation and a wider public will serve to hammer out a specific self-understanding of the occupation that allows it to be accepted as a profession. The purpose of this chapter is to explore this process of negotiation through an historical example, that of the artist in eighteenth-century Britain.

It will be suggested that, despite superficial indications to the contrary, the eighteenth-century artist is a typical professional. He will defend his professional status on the grounds that painters are primarily intellectuals. All that grinding of pigments and arduous manual labour in front of the canvas is beside the point. A history of painting may be construed as a story of technical and intellectual progress, with the scientific, professionally trained modern painter enjoying and exploiting the fruits of that development. As a profession, painting shares in and contributes to the Enlightenment's faith in reason and the perfectibility of humanity. Yet, as a profession, painting is also conservative. The appeal to rationality as a justification of the professional status and excellence of painting is balanced by an appeal to custom and tradition. Professional artists cannot afford to offend their clients, and a purely rational approach to painting may well be offensive.

It is precisely at this point, where there is a tension between reason and tradition, or between the universal and the parochial or subjective, that aesthetic values emerge as the overt focus of conflict and negotiation. The negotiation of the professional status of the painter is also a negotiation of the values that determine good art. It is a matter of taste. The conflict, however, is a deeper and ultimately political one, as to who determines what good taste is. The impolite or offensive painter (and we will meet one,

William Blake, in the course of this exploration) will not merely fail to sell paintings, they will fail to be accepted as a member of polite society, which is to say, of the middle classes. Thus negotiation of one's professional status is also a negotiation of one's class position. The painter only becomes a professional if they are accepted as a member of the polite middle classes. This entails that one submits the defining values of one's profession to public scrutiny and criticism. The contention, to be briefly outlined in the conclusion to this chapter, is that this negotiated class status is fundamental to all professions.

Painting and the bourgeois audience

A fundamental change occurred in European art from the late seventeenth to the late eighteenth centuries. This change is concerned not so much with matters of style as with the way in which art is understood and discussed. It is fundamentally the period in which the fine or beautiful arts are distinguished from those that are practical or mechanical. On one side stand sculpture, painting, music, poetry and dance. On the other there are useful activities, such as pottery, carpentry and metal work. Within this classification the fine arts are not useful, but they are important. Indeed, in the seventeenth century, their practitioners are beginning to aspire to a social status that would place them well above the artisans who practise the useful arts. How can something of no practical use be so exalted?

The forms of reflection on the visual arts that emerged in the eighteenth century respond to this conundrum. Many of the writings on art up to the seventeenth century concerned practical matters, reflecting upon the means of artistic execution, not its ends. By focusing on manual skills such as paint grinding, as well as the more refined techniques of representation and composition that were required by the artist, they emphasise the hard physical labour that is entailed in painting and sculpture (Harrison *et al.* 2000: 14). Thus they suggest that painters belong amongst the artisans. Although they may be respected, they remain 'Mechanicks'. However, with the rise of a newly educated and increasingly leisured middle class in the seventeenth and eighteenth centuries, there emerged a new pressure to reflect upon the purposes of art.

The middle class potentially represented a new source of livelihood for the artist, through a commercial market feeding bourgeois consumption. This market could compensate for the decline in church and state patronage. Yet, the task that lay before the artist was a complex one. Paintings and sculptures could not be sold to the middle class before its members had been convinced that this was the sort of thing in which they should take an interest. Painting and sculpture had served a purpose for the feudal state and church. For example, religious paintings might educate, encourage or intimidate congregations, and in addition display the power of the church. It was not evident that art could serve the same purpose, or indeed any purpose at all, for the middle class. The most obvious purpose that it might serve – that of decoration or entertainment – might be beneath its elevated consideration.

Perspectives on art

Early in the eighteenth century, the essayist Addison had begun to defend the contemplation of beauty on the grounds that it was an act of imagination. On the one hand, his argument is psychological, insofar as he situates imagination between the base senses and the higher faculty of reason. On the other hand, it is political. The place and status of the contemplation of beauty is determined in terms of class. He appeals to the fundamental eighteenth-century distinction between the 'polite' and the 'vulgar'. He notes that a 'man of polite imagination is let into a great many pleasures that the vulgar are not capable of receiving' (Addison 2000: 383). The exercise of the imagination is commended precisely because it appeals to the higher intellectual and moral aspirations of polite society.

Addison is concerned primarily with the contemplation of natural beauty. Richardson, a practising artist, is explicitly concerned to recommend the contemplation and patronage of art to the genteel. He notes the obvious problem that the arts seem only to produce 'pleasant Ornaments, mere Superfluities', but then defends art through the recommendation of a 'new science' of connoisseurship. He suggests that art is 'More Difficult, More Curious and More Beautifull than is Commonly Imagin'd' (Richardson 2000b: 332). In particular, although painting is grounded in the imitation of nature, Richardson claims that it is not mere mechanical imitation, but rather a rational and selective process that improves upon nature. It encourages and communicates an understanding of nature that could not be achieved otherwise. It thereby contributes to the process 'whereby Mankind advanced higher in the Rational State'. Again, painting appeals above the merely sensuous towards intellectual rewards.

David Hume poses the problem of art from a slightly different perspective (Hume 1996). Like Addison, Hume writes as a spectator rather than as a practitioner. His problem is not to justify polite interest in art as such, but rather to determine how the polite should judge and evaluate art. As Habermas observes, the eighteenth-century audience for art was unique, not just in its leisure and learning, but also in terms of the kind of art it consumed (Habermas 1989: 43–56). Crucially, the art consumed had been produced recently. Previously, if one read, one would typically read the classics. The status and excellence of the classics is never in doubt; the status of a new work is.

Hume addresses this concern by examining the possibility that there is a universal standard by which taste could be assessed and trained. Unfortunately, such a standard seems not to exist. Hume begins his essay by pointing to the 'great variety of taste, as well as of opinion, which prevails in the world' (Hume 1996: 133). There is a danger that in judging a work of art, one judges it purely on the grounds of the subjective pleasure that it yields. Judgements will be based upon what Hume calls 'sentiments', and '[all] sentiment is right; because sentiment has a reference to nothing beyond itself, and is always real, whenever a man is conscious of it' (Hume 1996: 136).

This is to say that if the worth of a work of art rested entirely upon subjective responses to it, then there would be no point in debating art. I like what I like; you like what you like. This would not merely undermine the possibility of art being a topic for polite conversation. More fundamentally, it would push the whole value and status of art back to merely sensual responses, making a nonsense of the new science of the connoisseur. Art would be no more than ornament and superfluity.

Hume responds by recognising the possibility of the existence of a standard of taste, but believes that few have developed the competence to recognise it. He identifies a series of judgements upon which people do agree. From this hint that there may indeed be commonly agreed judgements, he argues that it is incumbent on what Richardson would call a connoisseur to refine and develop the delicacy of their taste. Through this refinement the imperfections and prejudices of subjective judgement can be removed.

The process of refinement requires that would-be connoisseurs expose themselves to as many examples of art as possible and then employ reason to compare these works. The gross effects that may impress the novice are recognised for their lack of subtlety and refinement by the expert. Rational argument about taste then becomes possible, for refined judgement requires consistency. Subjective judgements are thus disciplined and made consistent through education and reason.

The implication is that the vulgar will remain at the level of purely subjective and particular judgements. Yet, more profoundly, Hume acknowledges that the ordinary member of polite society does not necessarily rise to the level of the connoisseur. The connoisseur is indeed a rarity. Even the polite require critics of refined and delicate taste to guide them. This raises the 'embarrassing' question of how one is to recognise a connoisseur (Hume 1996: 148). In effect, debate about the merits of a particular art work are displaced into even more fundamental debates about the merits of the critic who commends the work, and upon whom the polite art lover comes to rely to guide and educate their taste.

The importance of the critic

Hume's brief comments on the critic are of the utmost significance. On the one hand, they establish an important point about art. The merits of an art work are never obvious. A special refinement is required to evaluate art. On the other hand, it may be noted that Hume has said nothing about the social status of the artist. Hume seems to be indifferent to the possibility of regarding the painter as a mere mechanical. He is concerned with the status of the critic. The reason for this is simple. The good critic will be a member of polite society. They are fellow conversationalists. As such, they are professionals, for they have middle class status. The activity of critics is thus far more fundamental than the activity of artists.

In sum, while the likes of Addison, Richardson and Hume may have established art as something in which the middle class could take a serious interest, and indeed have established art as a topic for polite conversation, nothing has yet established that the artist is the social equal of the connoisseur. The aspiration to this status, and thus to what may be seen as the professionalisation of the artist, is expressed in the life, works and writings of Sir Joshua Reynolds.

Reynolds and the professionalisation of painting

Richardson observes that 'tis not every Picture-Maker that ought to be called Painter, as every Rhymer, or Grubstreet Tale Writer is not a Poet, or Historian: A Painter ought to be a Title of Dignity' (Richardson 2000a: 331). A 'Picture-Maker' may be a mere artisan or 'Mechanick', and would be so classified on the grounds that their trade entails the use of manual dexterity alone. The laborious nature of artistic production has been noted above, and could not be denied. Richardson therefore sought to defend the status of the painter by presenting it as the perfection of a manual skill, complemented by intellectual abilities, including an extensive knowledge of 'Anatomy, Osteology, Geometry, Perspective, Architecture', and in the case of the portrait painter 'an understanding of Mankind' and the ability to 'Think like a Gentleman' (in order to understand their subjects). The painter is therefore at once 'Curious Artificer' and an intellectual (Richardson 2000a: 331).

Sir Joshua Reynolds, painter and founder president of the Royal Academy of Arts, follows a similar line of argument. The annual *Discourses* that he presented to the Academy did much to define the status of the eighteenth-century painter, not least through reflection upon their training and education at the Academy (Reynolds 1975). His fourth discourse begins with the following proposition:

> The value and rank of every art is in proportion to the mental labour employed in it, or the mental pleasure produced by it. As this principle is observed or neglected, our profession becomes either a liberal art or a mechanical trade.
>
> (Reynolds 1975: 45)

Reynolds seeks for the artist what would now be understood as professional status. Crucially, artists can take their place in polite society because they are primarily intellectuals (despite possible obvious indications to the contrary).

In his second discourse, Reynolds proposes three stages to the training of an artist. There is an initial stage in which the student learns the basic mechanical skills required of the artist, including 'a facility of drawing any object that presents itself, a tolerable readiness in the management of colour, and acquaintance with the most simple and obvious rules of composition' (Reynolds 1975: 25). The second stage develops the student's theoretical knowledge. This may be seen to involve various elements. Nature (including human nature) is studied through a process of comparison that allows the artist to become aware of the ideal forms to which nature aspires, as opposed to the particular and defective forms it actually takes. The student should not learn to imitate nature mechanically, but rather to engage with it intellectually, in order to discover its beauty.

In the same way, and even more importantly, art history is studied. The student learns through imitation and comparison of the works of old masters exactly what their strengths and weaknesses are. Mere imitation is insufficient as that would involve a purely mechanical process. Rather, the student is being inducted into 'long converse with the greatest minds'. He or she enters into polite conversation with the artists of the past to develop a capacity, not merely to recognise their greatness but also their defects. Only when these stages of 'subjection and discipline' are complete is the artist able to proceed to the final stage of genuine creativity and the exercise of genius. Genius, Reynolds notes, begins 'where known vulgar and trite rules have no longer any place' (Reynolds 1975: 97).

Reynolds' overall purpose is clear. The artist is to undergo a refinement of taste similar to that required of Hume's critic. The goal of artistic training is to constrain the imagination of the artist within the discipline of sound mechanical technique and rationally justifiable rules of taste. Only when so constrained will imagination be fruitful. Artists gain their right to enter polite society on the grounds that they must be capable of exactly the same intellectual discernment and self-discipline as the critic or connoisseur.

Where Hume spoke of a 'standard of taste', Reynolds speaks of the fully trained artist 'comparing no longer the performances of Art with each other, but examining the Art itself by the standard of Nature', with 'Nature' here being taken to refer to nature perfected in the light of reason (Reynolds 1975: 27). The process of refinement of critic and artist may therefore be seen to be similar, in that it rests upon a reflective study of a canon of great artists. The artist goes beyond the critic only in that they do not merely reflect upon past works, but respond to them in their own work.

There is here already a vital move in the process of professionalisation. It was a move that was bitterly contested by the emerging generation of Romantic artists. William Blake's remarks written on his own copy of the *Discourses* make the point eloquently. The contention between Blake and Reynolds rests in their opposed conceptions of 'genius'. For Reynolds, genius is acquired through the training that disciplines the imagination. Blake conversely exalts original genius, believing that genius cannot be acquired but is innate in a few gifted individuals. Thus, Blake writes at the head of the seventh discourse:

> The Purpose of the following discourse is to Prove That Taste & Genius are not of Heavenly Origin & that all who have supposed that they Are so, are to be Consider'd as Weak headed Fanatics.
>
> (Blake 1975: 312)

Yet the dispute is not just about the nature of genius. Blake's original genius serves to undermine the professional status of the artist that Reynolds has fought to establish. If artists have original genius, then they serve them-selves and not a clientele. Their work will not be realised with rules that the client would recognise and appreciate. More problematically, if taste, too, is original rather than acquired, then the middle class cannot even be educated into appreciating that art. Blake thereby disrupts both the commer-cial basis of art and its place in polite society. Blake's art can give no guar-antee that it will not offend against politeness.

Reynolds must, in his own way, confront the problem posed by Blake's Romantic impoliteness. The disciplines that lead to the acquisition of genius must be acceptable to polite society. If a study of the history of art is at the core of this acquisition, then the way in which that history is understood is at stake.

As Reynolds notes, a diversity of models and exemplars clamour for the student's attention. Not all these models will serve the student well. The student must then ask upon whom they can rely, in order to lead them to genius.

Reynolds's initial answer is simple: 'those great masters' whose works 'have stood the test of ages'. Reynolds is therefore proposing, as a seemingly unproblematic task, the construction of a historical canon of great masters. But the assumption that a canon can be grounded merely on the seemingly empirical criterion of standing the 'test of ages' is disingenuous, and Reynolds recognises this. The canon does not select itself. Good and bad alike have survived, and good and bad alike may remain popular. The canon that Reynolds seeks to present to students is a history. Like all histories, it entails selection and evaluation.

It is, therefore, legitimate to ask after the fundamental aesthetic values that determine this process of selection and evaluation. Reynolds himself in fact debates at length who should be included and why (Reynolds 1975: 83–90). In principle, the debate might be resolved by appeal to the universal standard of taste. It is, however, precisely such a rational justification of the canon that can lead to the return of Blake's impoliteness. On the one hand, Reynolds has already been seen to emphasise that mere imitation is not of value to the artist. Appeal to nature and the canon alike presupposes the application of reason to assess the defects that inevitably lie in the model. This appeal to the universality of reason serves as a further justification of painting as a profession, for the canonical history of painting may be seen as the objective progress of the art to its present degree of perfection.

Painting is akin to medicine or law in that it can be gradually refined (and indeed, like medicine tested against nature and, like law, tested by the rational consistency of the judgements it makes). In looking back on the history of painting, the student comes to understand and to practise the perfections that their predecessors have achieved.

On the other hand, Reynolds, like Addison, Richardson and Hume, has suggested that painting is worthy of the attention of the middle class precisely because its value is not obvious. It requires a certain training and discernment to appreciate it. A problem emerges in the possibility that Reynolds' training programme is beginning to put that power of discernment beyond the scope of his middle class clientele. Unwittingly, Reynolds' professional is pushed into the position of Blake's Romantic genius. If the standard of taste (and thus adoption into the canon) rests entirely upon reason, then it may potentially offend the existing taste of the client.

Reynolds himself gives a fine example in the seventh discourse:

> There was a statue made not long since of Voltaire, which the sculptor, not having that respect for the prejudices of mankind which he ought to have, has made entirely naked, and as meagre and emaciated as the original is said to be. The consequence is what might be expected; it has remained in the sculptor's shop, though it was intended as a public ornament and a public honour to Voltaire, as it was procured at the expense of his contemporary wits and admirers.
>
> (Reynolds 1975: 140)

The sculptor may have been able to justify his work rationally, but it still runs against customary taste or prejudice, and thereby becomes absurd. This begins to throw into question the inviolability of a rational standard of taste.

The appeal to a standard of taste suggests that those who survive in the canon do so because they have not succumbed to the fluctuations of prejudice or custom. Elsewhere, Reynolds is less dismissive of custom (Reynolds 2000: 536–7). He suggests that one finds certain forms beautiful, not because of reason, but because of familiarity. We have become accustomed to the things we call beautiful. Reynolds reflects that if an Ethiopian were asked to paint the Goddess of Beauty, he would of course give her the typically Ethiopian features that would fall outside the European conception of beauty. On this account, the European view is merely different, not superior. This possibility is developed in the seventh discourse.

Reynolds initially seems to defend a standard of taste, arguing that prejudice is to be associated with 'apparent truth' as opposed to 'real truth'. An art that catered to such apparent truth would give mere pleasure, not instruction. Reynolds warns artists of too readily adapting their art to the tastes of the vulgar. The seventh discourse proceeds, however, to modify this argument. Reynolds suggests that long-standing prejudices may approach closely to truth, and distinguishes these from 'narrow' prejudices. In effect, this is to suggest that certain prejudices have a weight of tradition lying behind them, and more profoundly, that it is precisely this weight of tradition that embodies the progress of the arts. The artist can now be recommended to submit their own opinions to the discipline of the 'public voice'.

Reynolds's point is simple. The polite artist must hold their imagination in check, protecting it from the vulgarities of ornament and mere sensual pleasure on the one side, and from idiosyncratic invention (including the overzealous employment of reason) on the other. Only then can they aspire to the kind of genius that will secure for them a place in polite society.

Reynolds's approach to the professionalisation of the artist is highly conservative. The appeal to tradition and custom reinforces that conservatism, albeit under the guise of politeness. Artists established their professional status, on the one hand, by constructing an ideal to which their clientele are supposed to aspire – which is to say, Richardson's genteel connoisseur. Vulgar taste should have no influence over the artist. On the other hand, professional status is secured only insofar as the artist is allowed into the same social circles as the client. That demands of them politeness and a willingness to engage in polite conversation with the client and never simply to dictate to the client. An appeal to the objectivity of nature or reason, that might ground the doctor's or lawyer's paternalistic attitude towards their client, at least in the eighteenth century, is undermined from the start.

It may be noted that a consequence of this is that the very understanding of what it is to be an artist, which is to say, an understanding of the history of one's own profession, lies not in the artist's own hands, but again, in the results of conversation with the critic and the client.

Conclusion

These reflections on the eighteenth-century professionalisation of the painter have specific implications for how professions are understood in the twenty-first-century. Reynolds' approach to professionalisation highlights a series of paradigmatic qualities of professions. Professionals are primarily mental labourers. This is relatively unproblematic, but consideration of the case of painting does suggest that professionalism depends much upon the class aspirations of the practitioner, rather than specifically upon the type of activity involved.

Professions are conservative. Again, this is not an unexpected result. In part this conservatism may be expressed in and articulated by the stories that the professions tell of themselves, and crucially, the stories into which students are inculcated. Stories of professional heroes and villains (the Nightingales and Brunels, the Shipmans and Sarah Gamps) parallel

Reynolds' canon of great artists. What is problematic, however, are the criteria that are appealed to in order to construct such histories. Superficially it might be suggested that the heroes of medicine are, unproblematically, the great benefactors. The heroes of law may be similarly wise and beneficent. Put otherwise, in the language of Enlightenment progress, medical benefactors are testing themselves against nature. They bring about an improvement in health. Benefactors in law may be judged according to the rational consistency and brilliance of their understanding of legal tradition.

Painting could not appeal to such unambiguously pragmatic criteria, not least because the utility and worth of painting was radically uncertain in the eighteenth century. This brings into question the nature of innovation in any profession. It was suggested that painting was confined by the need to negotiate the nature of the profession with its clientele. Aesthetic values, broadly understood in terms of the need for politeness, displaced the objectivity of either mechanical imitation or intellectual rational analysis. Painting might then be seen to be a special case. It is apparently special, not simply because of the problematic nature of painting, but also because of the painter's clientele.

Professional painting constructs its clientele out of precisely the class to which the painter wishes to belong. The painter in addition seems to be special, because they cannot afford to be paternalistic (or at least their paternalism must be kept under tight rein). Once values that are wholly inherent to the activity of painting are placed at the core of the activity, as is done by Blake and the Romantics, painting ceases to be a profession.

The peculiarity of painting as a professional activity may only be apparent. While the twenty-first-century doctor or lawyer may be expected to take clients from all social strata, this was not obviously the case in the eighteenth century (Porter 1997: 255–8, 281–7). If the professional doctor was the physician who treated polite patients (and one might hazard, polite illnesses), then a high-handed paternalism, akin to Blake's disdain for his audience, was not an option. Just as the professional painter's appeal to reason had to be checked by custom in the name of politeness, similarly, it may be suggested, the defining values of the physician or lawyer could not just be those of the scientific Enlightenment. The medical and legal professions were as confined by the requirements of politeness as painting. The heroes of the profession are, again, not merely the rationally innovative, but also the polite.

Significantly, this entails, first, that specialist knowledge in medicine or the law did not serve to raise the eighteenth-century professional above their clients. Second, specialist scientific knowledge could not serve to justify paternalism. Paternalism would have been offensive. The particular treatment of a client would therefore have to be negotiated, and indeed the very values of the profession itself would be subject to public scrutiny.

It may be suggested that professional paternalism became problematic only in the twentieth century, precisely because of the changing class structure of Western societies. An initial expansion of the professional clientele to include all strata of society may have briefly allowed the legitimation of professional paternalism through expert knowledge (which perhaps marks a late triumph of the Enlightenment). As the middle classes expanded, paternalism increasingly came to be seen as problematic. The twenty-first-century professional therefore, ironically, finds themselves thrown back into the position of their eighteenth-century predecessor. Superior technical knowledge no longer allows the professional to be impolite to the client. If this is so, then not merely must the professional negotiate the details of an individual treatment with the client, but further questions about the nature and value of professions must be debated within society as a whole. The fate of the profession of the painter in the eighteenth century is not then a mere historical curiosity, but rather a paradigm of professionalisation and moral acceptable relationship of the professional to the client and wider public.

CHAPTER 4

The clergy: an interesting anomaly

Paul Ballard

Introduction

It was in the nineteenth-century that the professions, as we now recognise them, emerged as a powerful characteristic of our specialised, bureaucratic, technological, modern society. In our own day, however, there has been a real and far-reaching change in the esteem and freedom given to professional bodies as they have had to respond to political and cultural pressures. It is no surprise, therefore, that the professions have been of considerable sociological interest, both in themselves and as part of the wider social structures (Larson 1977; Abbott 1988; Macdonald 1995).

The clergy have long been regarded, along with medicine and law, as one of the classic learned professions. They, too, have attracted their own share of attention (Ranson *et al.* 1977; Towler and Coxon 1979). Such studies reveal both the parallels with, and differences from, other professional groups. For a number of reasons the clergy can be regarded as 'eccentric' (off centre). It is this that makes them of interest to those concerned with the nature and place of values in the professions. Through an illustrative selection of aspects of the profession, some key issues can be highlighted that are of significance for all professions.

A preliminary point must be made about the parameters of the ensuing discussion. The issues considered may indeed be widely found, but the case study has to be limited. Reference is, by and large, to the English context, except for the occasional cross-reference or inference. Even within such a confine there are variations and differences, most notably between the traditions characterised as Anglican, Nonconformist or Free Church Protestant and Roman Catholic. Inevitably, the established Church of England will dominate the story. To work on a wider canvas would require including too many variables and complexities for a short chapter.

The rise and decline of a profession

In many villages up and down the land the Old Rectory, or sometimes the Manse, is an imposing, desirable private residence. Meanwhile, the vicar or minister lives in a modest house across the green or even in the former garden. The older house, usually Georgian or Victorian, represents the high point of the socio-economic status of the clergy. It was in the eighteenth century that the clergy emerged as a learned profession and the pattern of ministry that was until recently assumed to be normal was established. The parson had become part of the establishment, albeit often somewhat lowly, but even the poorer clergy were not unusually well educated and no longer effectively farmers of smallholdings (Russell 1980).

This development was, however, part of that process of differentiation that was increasingly to characterise modern society. In mediaeval Christendom the clergy had been a religious class, with the Pope at its head and its own structures and laws, parallel to the secular arm of the King and the nobility. Moreover, the clergy provided for not only the religious but also the learned needs of society: education, administration and welfare.

From the fifteenth and sixteenth centuries, however, parallel to the emergence of the modern state, mercantilism and science, specialised social functional structures emerged and went their separate ways. The clergy were no less part of this process. The Reformation had radically redefined the relation between Church and state. The minister or priest was seen as primarily having a pastoral and liturgical function, though only slowly shedding the educational and welfare aspects. Over time, too, these functions were also taken over by the state so that the clergy's activity became increasingly circumscribed.

At the same time the Protestant demand for a learned clergy and the Catholic Tridentine (Counter-Reformation) model of priesthood called for professional specialised practice that demanded training. Out of this emerged the theological college or seminary – even though in Anglicanism this only really happened in the nineteenth century (Day 1979; Hastings 1987). Yet the narrow professionalisation of the clergy within the religious realm or community has never been wholly complete. Up to the present they have always been seen as community leaders – because of their presence on committees and at communal functions – and not simply as religious functionaries. Also, unlike most other occupational groups, many clergy have always had jobs that are not directly linked with their ordination: for example, in the ecclesial institution as administrators or advisors, or in secular employment as teachers. Today this has increased with the widespread ordination of part-time and non-stipendiary clergy. There is not necessarily a simple correspondence between ordination and employment.

Nevertheless, the situation today is very different from the times of Jane Austen and Anthony Trollope. We hear of livings made up of several parishes, lack of recruitment, financial stringency and clergy stress (Church Information Office 1985 and 1990; Coate 1989). Increasingly, despite a residual social eminence, the clergy appear to be comparatively margina-lised. Furthermore, many clergy are not trained for full-time ministry in a limited number of universities and they earn their living by undertaking non-ecclesiastical employment, so they undertake clerical work essentially as part-time volunteers. This suggests that in many ways they are becoming de-professionalised in conventional terms (Pattison 1989: 153ff). This change, which has occurred most rapidly since the 1960s, is instructive and germane to other professional groups. The reasons for it can be broadly set out under three headings.

The secularisation process

The first factor is contextual. A profession depends on its cultural accept-ability. If there is indifference or scepticism then decline sets in. For the clergy this can be understood in terms of what is meant by 'secularisation' (Lyon 1985; Davie 1994, 2000; Bruce 1996; Hunt 2002). The process described in the previous section left the clergy as the religious experts. This is possible to sustain when society, officially and in practice, understands the Church as a focal institution, embodying its values and beliefs. But if this ceases to be the case, the clergy find themselves pushed to the edge of society and increasingly working within the confines of the community of faith, which itself has become a voluntary optional organisation. Thus they are caught between trying to sustain their public role – often by moving into areas such as counselling, teaching or chaplaincy – or accepting the limita-tions of the institutional boundaries of the Church. In a pluralistic and open market they are driven to struggle for recognition (Towler and Coxon 1979).

The plurality of traditions

A second factor is that at least since the Reformation, there has never been a religious monopoly. The attempt to impose an Anglican settlement had collapsed by the end of the seventeenth century. Nonconformity and Catho-licism steadily won equality of status so that today the three traditions regard themselves, more or less, as partners. Unlike other professions, there-fore, the clergy never had an exclusive monopoly guaranteed by the state. And even within the Church of England there were party conflicts. Indeed, Anglicanism has made a virtue of being the *via media*, a bridge between the different traditions (Neill 1977; Avis 1989; Sykes *et al.* 1998).

The changed relationship between clergy and lay people

Thirdly, there has been within the churches, especially through the latter half of the twentieth century, a movement to understand the Church in corporate rather than hierarchical terms. This can best be illustrated by reference to the changes within the Catholic Church at and since the Second Vatican Council (1963–65). The Church is widely understood as a 'pilgrim people' and 'the body of Christ'; the liturgy is now in the vernacular with more participation by the congregation; there is an emphasis on a personal exploration of belief; and above all there is stress on the active place of the laity. Similar moves can be found in almost every Christian tradition. The result is to blur the distinction between clergy and laity. In the spirit of the age the professional is not assumed to be the sole repository of excellence or authority (Butler 1981; Flannery 1981; Hastings 1991).

The clergy, therefore, have experienced in a radical way the current collapse of the professional mystique. There is ambiguity, however, as there is in all change. The problem is that a desire for new values can weaken older, but no less important, values. For instance, collegiality that attempts to engender professional responsibility can sometimes lead to some clergy being marginalised or excluded. Yet, if attempts are made to rectify this in the name of accountability by, for example, minimising boundaries, this change may perhaps produce a lesser sense of responsibility in a situation open to greater litigation.

The monopoly over knowledge and practice is challenged. Values like trust and authority have been eroded and have to be renegotiated. Custom and tradition, which can provide a liberating security but which can also lead to professional sclerosis, have been overtaken by a continuous suspicion and experimentation, which can be both challenging and destructive. Moreover, where the structures shake loose the response tends to be bureaucratic and technological. This is not the best way to build a sense of common community and enterprise.

Representative persons

Religion is far from dead. A significant proportion of the population still turns up at the vicarage door requesting a religious rite of passage – 'hatches, matches and despatches'; or, in an age of pluralism, they can go elsewhere or call on their own expressions of 'spirituality'. Again, national and civic events, such as Remembrance Day or a Jubilee or a lament for a dead princess or a Hillsborough disaster, are led or attended on by clergy, possibly including those from other 'faith communities'.

Some may suggest these are expressions of a fading past. Yet it seems that society always needs symbolic expressions of its own self-understanding and place in the mystery and depth of existence. In an age of transition, part of the uncertainty is whether and how these symbols and perceptions are to be reworked. The clergy, however, are still widely regarded as symbolic figures, representing and mediating essential social perspectives and values (Bocock and Thompson 1985; McGuire 1987; Parsons 2002).

It is not surprising, therefore, to find that discussions of the theoretical foundations on which they base their authority make almost no reference to professional criteria. The starting point is theological; that is, the relation-ship believed to pertain between God and the universe as creator and saviour and how this informs what it means to be human (Commission on Faith and Order 1982; Hall and Hanniford 1996; Croft 1999). The ministry is there to represent the values that are understood to 'shape our ends' and to serve these ends through the life of the Church and in the wider society. Like any other profession, the clergy are there to offer a public service. But the point to be underlined here is that in this case this service is referred back to a more fundamental set of questions about human meaning and purpose and how the professional activity serves and reflects the wider good and human values. These are questions that are probably not widely discussed in the professions, although the quest to create ethical statements and codes of practice must surely relate to such issues.

In the modern or post-modern context, where there is little consensus, metaphysical questions about the nature of human good are difficult to handle. Yet they will not go away and are necessary if particular activ-ities are to be part of the common life. What are the aims to which this or that activity is committed? How does it promote human well-being? From whence are such values derived? Are they invented or drawn from fundamental given realities (Holmes 1978)? The professional person, therefore, has to take on board that they not only represent their profes-sion's expertise and integrity but are working on a wider stage and partly responsible for society as a whole, representing and sustaining its values and welfare.

Vocation and formation

The previous discussion leads to another distinctive emphasis on what it means to be a clergy person. In the selection and training of ministers, primacy is given to their inner personal development. This is because it is assumed that the task of the clergy is bound up with a way of life and a quality of being. This is illustrated by the way the clergy, as with other public exemplars, are pilloried in the media at any hint of scandal. The heart of pastoral practice and spiritual leadership is not simply providing a service, but a relationship with people in their daily lives as they travel on their own personal pilgrimage struggling with the difficulties and burdens of life. This dimension can be briefly illustrated in two ways.

People commonly talk about a 'vocation' to the priesthood or ministry. By this is meant a sense of direction and rightness that makes taking up such a profession feasible. It is less about choosing a career and more like commit-ting oneself to a cause. Part of the induction process is to have that 'call' tested and affirmed (or challenged). This provides the motivation for sustaining a career that can often be undertaken in straightened or lonely circumstances. This does not, however, have to be understood in highly mystical terms or as a 'Damascus road' experience. Nor ought it be thought of as unique to the clergy or other religious such as missionaries or nuns. In fact, in the Protestant tradition which has informed British culture, each and every occupation can properly be called a vocation, paid or unpaid, with its sense of rightness and commitment (Whipp 1997).

Yet some occupations have always had a stronger sense of vocation, especially those providing a public caring service – doctors, nurses, social workers, teachers – but fire fighters, aid workers and others could also be included. In a real sense one can be 'engaged' or betrothed to a profession. Indeed the word vocation suggests the act of taking up a way of life that is comprehensive and inclusive, often, traditionally, by taking a vow, as with the Hippocratic oath in medicine. But in our age of individualism and public accountability, where there is a fairly sharp distinction between the public arena of work and the private, personally controlled life of home and leisure, such a model may seem archaic and restrictive. However, it can be argued that this sense of commitment is an essential element in human society, making for reliability and community, and that this is especially true of the professions (Whipp 1997).

Complementary to a sense of vocation is the idea of 'formation'. The training of a priest or minister is not so much acquiring technical knowledge and skills (though this is clearly important), nor even the development of 'people skills' (though these are indispensable). Nor is the ordinand setting out on a career (though there can be preferment). The clergy person is entering into a way of life. So time is given to inculcating certain qualities of being, to developing a 'spirituality' in their own personal preparation (Ramsay 1985). Again, rather than concentrating on the technical and functional, perhaps such an emphasis ought to be included in most, if not all, professional training, even if there is never any guarantee of total success.

This sense of vocation and process of formation for the professional practice of ministry tends to be at odds with current attitudes. To be a priest or minister is to be a 'public person'. While there has to be a proper place for family, friendship and fun, there is never a complete escape from one's professional identity. The private and the public merge into one. The calling informs who one is.

Perhaps, however, the current stress on the separation between the public and private is more of an illusion than is often admitted, not least in professional life. That which occupies so much time and thought every day, carrying responsibility and dependent on high levels of training and reflective practice, is bound to shape those so engaged. This is almost certainly more so in professions that work in and with the community. Arguably, most professions as well as the public require more of their members in terms of commitment and personal involvement in their work than is recognised in formal contracts of employment or job descriptions. Whether justifiably or not, some caring professions have a notion of the perfect, complete professional, virtuous in all parts of their lives, implicit in their codes of practice (Pattison 2001; Edgar 2003).

The employers of non-caring professionals, such as accountants or archi-tects, also recognise the problem. Even if the law now does not allow it, they are often as interested in a person's psychological profile, social aptitudes and even family life as in his/her professional skills. Many professionals are finding that the demands of the job do not respect a neat division between corporate and private time as they juggle the demands of job and family in an age of increasing pressure.

Incidentally, this question is also posed by another way by which our lives tend to be separated out into segments: the physical distance between home and work through commuting. By contrast, the parson is often the only professional still living in the community they serve, especially among the urban poor. It was not long ago that others, such as the doctor, district nurse or teacher, were part of the community alongside the shopkeeper or postmistress. Attempts are made to reintegrate the community by, for example, health, advice or law centres; but they are still often serviced from outside.

All this raises the question about the nature of professional identity. What does it mean to be a doctor or a lawyer or engineer or bank manager? How do role and personality interrelate? In what sense is one a 'public person'? How do home, hobbies, family and other aspects of life shape professional commitment? And how does professional commitment affect the personal lives of professionals?

The professional amateur or court jester

One of the marks of a profession is that it practises its skill on the basis of the mastery of a body of knowledge that is held in trust for the laity that receive the service offered. The quality of service is guaranteed in the profes-sional identity. However, here too the clergy find themselves somewhat in a dilemma due to the nature of their vocation. Ironically, the clergy are precisely in the game of making available to others both the theoretical and practical knowledge they live by. The minister not only works alongside a whole range of lay ministries but seeks to induct people into the wisdom and practice of their faith. In a sense the parson can be regarded as the only professional seeking to work themselves out of a job.

It is not that there is no body of knowledge. As with any long-standing living tradition, Christianity has an immense body of literature, including its sacred scriptures, and a depth of practical wisdom and tradition. There are learned specialists, theologians and others engaged in reflection and study. But the aim is, in the end, to enable this wisdom to be accessible to all.

A similar point can be made about professional boundaries. This can be well illustrated in relation to hospitals and hospital chaplains. In tending the sick there is a team of experts, each with their specialised knowledge and skills, from the doctors and surgeons through the nursing staff, physiotherapists and social workers to the ward assistants and other support staff. The boundaries between different groups may be continuously under dispute as they jostle for prestige or new working practices are brought into play. But it is in this game that the chaplains have to find their place (Faber 1971).

The natural assumption is that the chaplain looks after the 'spiritual' dimension (though nurses are presently laying claim to cover this). The chaplain's task may not only include pastoral care but also some participation in ethical and other similar discussions. This would seem to agree with the professional perception of the clergy as the religious functionary, as outlined earlier (Dunstan 1967). This is currently a major preoccupation of those clergy in areas of healthcare as they adapt to new National Health Service (NHS) structures (Orchard 2001).

Yet there is in fact an alternative view possible. The chaplain can understand the task as not simply being there for the patient's religious needs, though that is a dominant care. They can consider the whole hospital as the parish and wish to become engaged with the whole enterprise, the values and meanings that inform healthcare itself, and how that is embodied in the conditions and relationships in which staff and patients find themselves.

The chaplain is, therefore, not a specialist but a generalist, someone with no natural home, and can use freedom given by the job to become informed and concerned, supporting, challenging and working alongside and with all those involved in the enterprise at every level. Demarcation boundaries in one sense fade away, though there would always be a proper recognition of others' expertise. In fact, it is to seek the freedom but also the risk of the margins. It has been likened to the court jester, the one who is present, trusted, yet without status; or described as the professional amateur, the one who is dedicated and skilled but not confined or specialised (Faber 1971). Other clergy are in a similar position; the parish priest alongside the general practitioner (GP), headteacher or the police and the industrial chaplain winning the respect of both unions and management (Melinsky 1992; Claringbull 1994; Dawn and Peterson 2000).

Conclusion

This paper has attempted to compare and contrast the clerical profession with the accepted ideal type of a profession as a self-regulating body, autonomous under the law, offering a public service on the basis of a recognised field of expertise and knowledge, with special reference to those points that raise questions about values. It would appear that the clergy do not fit this normative pattern. Indeed, there are many clergy who would want to argue that it is inappropriate to seek to describe themselves as a profession; or at least to use it in a highly qualified sense (Pattison 2000). It has been this tension that has been used to raise the questions about the source, place and nature of values among the professions in general.

Ironically there are signs, just when the professions are under considerable pressure to defend and modify their traditional social status, of new moves among the clergy to increase their sense of professionalism. This can be seen, for example, in the desire of some to revise their terms of employment (presently as self-employed) and to form some kind of professional association. There have also begun to appear a number of, mainly American, handbooks on ministerial ethics (Lebacqz 1985; Weist and Smith 1990; Wind *et al.* 1991; Chadwick 1994; Gula 1996). This is due to the need to establish an identity as well as the need to comply with increasing state regulation of employment. But the ambiguity of desiring professional status, while perceiving or experiencing the erosion of professional freedom, simply reflects what is happening in varying degrees across the whole professional spectrum, from the established through to the new and aspiring groups.

PART II

Value conflicts and professional identity

Introduction

Socially, we are what we do for a living. When we meet someone for the first time, a number of standard questions are commonly employed to establish who exactly we are talking to and what we might expect of them. This helps us to decide how best to relate to the stranger and manage any subsequent interaction. High up on the list comes a query along the lines 'And what do/did you do for a living?' Establishing how a person spends their working life enables us to make predictions about their social status, income, educational level, even their attitudes to social and political issues.

Work, particularly paid work, significantly determines how people conceive of, and react to, each other. It is crucial to our notions of ourselves and our identity. The *type* of work we do is especially relevant to our feelings of identity, self-esteem and the value we place on ourselves. Professional work is seen as providing greater job satisfaction and intrinsic reward than other routine employment. Professionals have the freedom (or autonomy) to control their own work; they make decisions involving the exercise of judgement based on their own particular expertise. In the case of the more traditional professions, the exercise of professional judgement has mainly been in relation to an individual client; hence the emphasis on the *nature* of the relationship between them.

As many codes of practice and statements from professional bodies bear witness, it is generally assumed that key values for professionals are autonomy, integrity and honesty. Provided that the professionals perceive themselves as implementing and upholding these values in their daily practice, they should feel that their work is worthwhile, enjoy job satisfaction and experience high self-esteem.

Problems will arise for the individual, however, if:

- strongly held personal values conflict with professional values
- the values of one profession are different from, and therefore potentially conflict with, the values of another occupational group in the same context
- the implementation of professional values is hindered by factors arising from the immediate organisational setting and other external exigencies.

In the contemporary world, many professionals no longer work in a simple one-to-one client relationship in businesses and premises that they own. Many work for salaries in managed public organisations alongside different kinds of professional groups. Often they are accountable in several different directions. They may have to cope with maintaining their own distinctive identity and values in a context which seems to demand considerable modification so that all professional groups fit in and work to a common purpose and ethos.

The following chapters all deal with the real tensions that arise in professional and personal values and identity in organisations. They approach this from the perspective of three recently emergent professional groups which are currently attempting to manage and reconcile their values in different institutional contexts in the United Kingdom (UK). These groups are all products of the increasing specialisation that has taken place among the occupations that provide services in the public sector. This specialisation has brought about the rise of many new and aspiring professions. All three examples illustrate professionals seeking to manage their values in an ever-changing environment.

The first chapter considers the situation of National Heath Service (NHS) managers. Should they attempt to emulate other professional groups within the health or public service sphere, or should they conceive of their role and identity differently? In a striking counter-example to the assumption that as occupational groups develop they will more or less inevitably seek professional status, values, etc., this chapter shows that an influential and skilled group may not always choose to become a profession in the formal, narrow sense. This is particularly the case if its values and practice have to accommodate situations and issues which go beyond the traditional professional–client relationship. In the case of leisure management professionals, the subject of the second chapter, what should the values and responsibilities of a newly emergent, slightly fragile occupational group be in relation to the complex social environment and decisions for which they are partly responsible? Finally, the example of social workers poses complex questions about how social workers might define and implement their values amidst the ambiguity of many of the sensitive issues and cases in which they are bound to intervene.

In Chapter 5 'Is health service management a profession?', Andrew Wall, a former NHS chief executive who now lectures and writes on health management policy, draws on his own experience to question whether or not it makes sense for NHS managers to conceive of themselves as professionals along the lines of other professional groups in health or public service. NHS managers work in a highly professionalised environment with 'tribes' of powerful, clinical, client-focused occupational groups which have very clear historical identities and values. Medicine is the most powerful of these groups. At the same time, managers are required to respond to the imperatives of political fiat and social need and are increasingly under central governmental control. Inevitably clinical, managerial and political values conflict, with managers having to negotiate their way through a mire of complexity and confusion.

In this context, it might make sense to opt for the clarity and solidarity that a professional role and body might provide with distinctive values, self-regulation, control of entry and exit to the profession and so on. This could enhance the effectiveness and confidence of members of the managerial occupational caste.

However, Wall points out that most managers do not seem to want this. Furthermore, the option for professional status modelled on clinical or public-servant professional paradigms might actually be a hindrance in pursuing their own distinctive function. So, in the end, Wall rejects the professional model and status as an unsuitable one for this occupational group. While the adjective 'professional' might loosely be used of NHS managers by themselves or others, he believes that they do not need, and should not aspire, to be a profession like other occupational groups within and outside the healthcare arena. This is a surprising conclusion in a social climate in which the bid for professional status seems to be regarded as a universal benefit by most occupational groups. Even without formal professional status, however, Wall points out there are considerable benefits in terms of status, self-esteem and power to being a senior NHS manager, even if the value tensions of life 'at the top' are considerable.

The evolving tensions between professional, managerial and political values are a central focus for the next chapter. Stephen Howell is a director of leisure services currently conducting postgraduate research on the role of leisure professionals. Michael McNamee is an applied philosopher with a special interest in sport and leisure. In Chapter 6 'Equity versus efficiency: managing competing values for the public sector leisure professional', Howell and McNamee discuss another example of a fundamental clash of values in a changing situation as leisure services managers (LSMs) attempt to define their role and function.

Howell and McNamee argue that it is their function as mediators and managers of the values implicit in central and local government directives and the views of local people and local politicians that underpins the LSM's claim to be 'professional', and not merely a local government employee. Having shown the inadequacy of a simple utilitarian approach in mediating between the public sector value of equity (fair shares of services for all) and the private sector value of efficiency (value for money) in the field of leisure provision, they stress the LSM's position as 'expert advisor'. As competent professionals, LSMs should, they believe, play an important part in informing the decisions of the local councillors, giving advice on the feasibility and efficiency of various options while taking into account local preferences and the overall distribution of resources within a fixed budget. Unfortunately, the changing nature of the leisure sector, with increasing involvement of charities and other bodies, raises considerable challenges for the emergent advisory role of the Client Officer, leaving the future of professional advice in the public leisure services unclear.

Ambiguity and lack of clarity characterise the role and function of professional social workers, as the third and final chapter in this part of the book shows. In Chapter 7 'Value dilemmas and social work practice', Jeremy Roche, an academic lawyer now teaching health and social welfare policy at the Open University, points up the complexities surrounding the changing role of those working in the personal social services. Unlike NHS managers and leisure service professionals, registered social workers have a very clear, articulate value base. This emphasises protecting the rights and promoting the interests of the client/service user, while at the same time protecting them as far as possible from danger or harm, and ensuring that their behaviour does not damage themselves or others. However, these clear values create the possibility of real conflict once professional social workers start to make decisions, determining judgements and interventions. Quite apart from their own personal values, their professional assessment of the situation and the priority accorded to different primary values can result in very different courses of action, leading to a lack of consensus and consistency in practice.

Such a lack of consensus in practice raises questions about the nature of the expertise being claimed, the values being enacted, and how judgement in decision making is structured. Since social workers are dealing with people who have problems in everyday life we are all 'experts' in this field, including the clients themselves. A complicating factor is that clients may be under some compulsion to accept the service offered rather than voluntarily seeking it out. Social work 'expertise' is thus much more likely to be challenged and come under scrutiny from clients and society as a whole than would be the case with lawyers or doctors – witness the high-profile cases of failure of social workers to intervene appropriately into which inquiries have been held.

Roche shows how social workers can find it very difficult to remain value-centred in their practice because of changes in the regulatory framework of law and wider expectations. Like the NHS managers, they are experiencing greater demands for accountability and pressure to have clearer rules and procedures. This limits their freedom to make decisions according to their best judgement. This represents a considerable challenge to professionally defined identity, role and values.

It is possible to highlight a number of general emergent themes and issues from all three chapters in this section.

First, *value conflict* is a very real issue in occupational groups as varied as NHS managers, social workers and LSMs. It is therefore likely to be significant in many other professions. It is probable that there will be obvious points of tension between the personal values an individual brings into a work situation – values that will differ according to past socialisation and experience by gender, ethnic group, class, religion, etc. – and the professional and organisational values that they may have to implement in everyday practice. Fundamental value conflict can exist within and between professions. There can also be a conflict between the values of professions and professionals and those of organisations and whole societies. This kind of conflict presents itself fairly sharply when professionals have to square professional and managerial values, a common situation when professionals of all kinds participate in organisations with their own values and purposes which transcend those of particular professions.

Secondly, the issue of value conflict raises the point that in complex modern societies and organisations it may be *very difficult to determine whose interests and values should be served by professionals*. Professionals have traditionally seen their main responsibility as being to their client(s), defending their interests and ensuring that their needs are met. Should professionals serve the needs of individual clients or those of their employing organisations? This, in turn, raises the broader issue of what exactly is the professionals' duty to the wider society? Is it appropriate for them to remain unaware or ignore the implications of their practice for the good of the community as a whole? Clearly, in the case of all the professions considered here, it would be perverse to take the view that professionals have no duty to society as a whole. However, this concession imperils the clarity of professional roles, duties and values in ways that may be very unhelpful in everyday practice unless it is recognised that perhaps an integral part of being a professional is to actively manage and make judgements in situations of value conflict.

Thirdly, it is worth noting that in professional work in the public sector there may well be *conflicts (both implicit and explicit) between the values of the public sector and those of the private sector*. Even within the former, values associated with the latter may creep in due to the adoption of private sector practices and assumptions associated with management. An interesting concept in this connection is that of the professional as 'mediator of values'. It might perhaps be an important part of the professional's expertise precisely to reconcile the values of the stakeholders with whom s/he is dealing. However, the difficulties of undertaking this kind of reconciliation or mediation on an everyday basis should not be underestimated – the strain it can impose on the individual professional is evident in these chapters.

A fourth emergent theme is that of the *rapidly changing nature of the roles, duties and values of professions*. NHS managers, LSMs and social workers are quite recent arrivals upon the professional scene. Even within the short time of their existence, these occupational groups have had to change, interpret and negotiate around their practices and values to cope with their changing environments with the many different demands and expectations that they bring. Responses vary considerably, from the social workers' clarity about core values and full embracing of a professional role and identity, to the NHS managers' ambivalence about identifying themselves as professionals with distinct values and expectations of occupational members. These responses are influenced by the nature of the work and function which each of these groups is required to perform. An implication is that one should not expect to see different occupational groups behaving in the same ways to deal with tensions in values. Indeed, there is a wide variety of possible means of coping with these tensions that would benefit from much greater attention and articulation.

CHAPTER 5

Is health service management a profession?

Andrew Wall

Introduction

Managers in the National Health Service (NHS) are in an unenviable position. Blamed by the public for administrative shortcomings, held to account by government for a bewildering number of targets and often derided by the clinicians with whom they work, it is surprising that this career is seen as attractive by anyone. Yet applications for the National Management Training Scheme, with an annual intake of 70 students, mostly new graduates, remain at a high level. From limited research as to what motivates these applicants, it appears that the job's variety, the level of responsibility and the opportunities for introducing change are the factors which most appeal, together with a desire to work in the public sector. This chapter will explore to what extent health service managers as public servants can claim to be seen as members of a profession and whether such a claim is relevant in their relationships with patients, clinical colleagues and the government.

The discussion is rooted in my considerable experience as a health service manager culminating in the 20 years when I held the chief managerial post of a health district providing services for a population of 400 000. The dearth of reflective accounts of what it is like to be a health service manager suggests that even one such manager's observations may be useful in the debate on the nature of public service in an increasingly compromised welfare state.

The rise in the importance of management has been a phenomenon of the last 50 years. This has been particularly evident in the NHS. In 1948, the NHS inherited several different styles of management. The old voluntary hospitals had been administered – the preferred word – by what might be called gentlemen amateurs. Their main duties were to maintain good relations with their local communities to ensure the continued financial viability of their hospital. The day-to-day operational aspects of the hospital were in the hands of the matron. Local authority hospitals were more likely to have a medical superintendent at their head with a steward, essentially a procurement and facilities manager, assisting. Community health services were under the control of each local authority's medical officer of health.

Gradually the administrators, in due course renamed managers, were perceived as becoming more necessary for the running of the NHS. In 1974, the introduction of consensus management placed the administrator as an equal on a team otherwise made up of professionals, three doctors, a nurse and an accountant. Their status was further elevated when the Griffiths report proposed that there should be one general manager at the top of each organisation (Department of Health and Social Security 1983). The majority of people appointed to this role were administrators. The 1990 Act, which introduced the internal market to the NHS, enhanced the apparent standing of the role of top manager with the title chief executive.

I have suggested elsewhere that the change of title from administrator to general manager and then to chief executive only acknowledged what had been evident for some years: the role of the top manager naturally put them in the position of *primus inter pares* because of the functions attached to the role (Wall 1999). Others have maintained that fundamentally the relative status of managers and clinicians has not changed (Harrison *et al.* 1992). Clinicians have sapiential authority enclosed within tight professional boundaries. This cannot be breached by managers, whose own professional status is questionable. Managers no doubt consider that they approach their work in a professional manner, that is, with demonstrable competence and with due concern for fairness and honesty. But those attributes are insufficient in themselves to confirm professional status.

Why should challenging NHS managers' professional status matter? Do managers themselves wish to be considered as members of a profession and, if so, how could they justify this claim? Management is a functional activity. Would professional status make any difference to what they do? Health service managers are public servants. How would professional status affect their relationships with the communities they serve or with the government to whom they are accountable?

NHS managers' view of themselves

Management in the NHS is undertaken by two main groups of people, those with a general management background and those initially trained as clinicians. Although the balance has changed in recent years, those with a general management background are more likely to hold the most senior posts. While some may have entered this line of work fortuitously where a situation arose and they applied and were successful (Dawson *et al.* 1995), others will have made a more considered choice. Evidence on their motivation is limited. One study indicated that in addition to the variety and the high level of responsibility, entrants wished to work specifically in the public sector (Wall 2001). It might, therefore, be assumed that what is often referred to rather vaguely as the 'public sector ethos' was an attraction, even if only negatively as a rejection of the commercialism of the private sector.

> It is an interesting, fast-moving world, socially worthwhile, useful.
> (Mike Fry in Wall 2001: 10)

> I couldn't get up in the morning and think about going and making toothpaste for a living, although some people do.
> (Heather Rice in Wall 2001: 10)

> I am in the NHS because I want to do something meaningful.
> (Jacqueline Myers in Cole 2002a: 10)

'Making a difference', 'helping people', 'not being concerned with profit' are all factors mentioned. Managers enjoy enhanced self-esteem because they see themselves as doing 'something worthwhile'. Despite the relatively negative perception of public service bureaucrats, they hope to receive some credit for their commitment to public welfare.

Working for the common good in providing worthwhile services for the community is often fundamental to managers' motivation. As they take on more senior jobs, they also show strong support for those managerialist principles more commonly associated with the private sector, such as target setting, value for money and efficiency.

Managers have also tried to modernise their perceptions of themselves. No longer do they wish to be merely enablers, providing an environment for clinical work. They want to prove that they are equal to their private sector colleagues, able to manage efficiently with a due regard for the 'bottom line' and to achieve stated goals within a strategic framework. The term 'administration', with its bureaucratic process-dominated associations, is no longer acceptable. After the Griffiths report in 1983, the following trends could be observed: making pay comparisons with the private sector a legitimate negotiating tool, the acceptance of short-term contracts and performance-related pay and less nervousness at holding meetings in expensive hotels. There was increasing emphasis on proactive management setting the strategic agenda and correspondingly less inclination to be reactively concerned with problem solving. Senior managers' behaviour became more like that of their private sector counterparts.

Despite this emulation of some of the attributes of private sector managers, there appears still to be a difference between them:

> Managers in the NHS were rated by their immediate subordinates
> ... more highly than their private sector counterparts in terms of
> interpersonal skills and intellectual ability and also on managing

change and an entrepreneurial approach – the dimensions strongly associated with the private sector.

(Alimo-Metcalfe and Alban-Metcalfe 2002: 27)

This flattering account does not mean that NHS managers necessarily feel comfortable. Having chosen to work in the public sector they experience considerable strain:

> I would like to make decisions about how the NHS is run. I'm concerned, though, at the increasing tendency to scapegoat managers for problems which are often deep-rooted and difficult to address in the timescales demanded.
>
> (Daniel Elkeles in Cole 2002a: 29)

Tensions and coping strategies among senior managers

With advancing seniority, the tensions for managers increase. Their sense of public service is put under greater strain by the exigencies of the job and by demands made upon them by government. There are dangers that their original motivation will become corrupted:

> People lose track of the fact that this is a public service and what we're not here for is self-aggrandisement. We need to be reminded regularly of why we're doing what we're doing
>
> (Neil Goodwin in Davies 2001: 23)

Notably, a significant number of top managers have left the NHS well before their expected retirement date. For some this has been a relief:

> I dread approaching a state of mind ... [when] what are personal blind spots become organisational weaknesses
>
> (Mike Fry in Wall 2001:16)

Most chief executives only have a certain amount they can give an organisation before it is time to move (Cole 2002b). Worryingly, few of those who have left the NHS seem to have any regrets about what they left behind. But for others the sense of loss continues:

> I still feel angry about what happened to me – two to three years is not long enough to get over something like that. It wasn't a job it was a way of life for me.
>
> (John Beecher in Snell 2000: 25)

At its simplest, all that may be being observed here is the natural history of growing older. The idealism of youth develops into a more grounded perception of reality where toleration of ambiguity and compromise are required if the aims of the organisation are to be fulfilled. Nevertheless, choice is still an option:

> ... if you feel you are being asked to bend too far then at that point you have to say "I cut my losses, and I leave and do something else"
> (Pam Charlwood in Wall 2001: 23)

But making a stand is self-limiting. Once out of job, you have no influence. If the manager is concerned, within their own perception and values, to affect outcomes, they may rationalise an ethical compromise on the grounds that it is better to accept a smaller evil to attain a greater good.

Several strategies can be employed here. The first is to lie low, knowing that everything passes and today's principal task rapidly becomes outdated. Some managers adopt a second, 'evangelical' approach, welcoming every new initiative with public support, extolling them as 'exciting', 'radical' and, above all, 'modern'. A third response is to comment anonymously through unascribed scepticism in the press or suitably generalised statements from a representative body such as a trade union or, in this case, the Institute of Healthcare Management (IHM). So in a report on the introduction of *The NHS Plan* (Department of Health 2000b), and its follow-up *Shifting the Balance* (Department of Health 2001), managers were quoted anonymously as saying:

> Governments never learn that reorganisations disrupt delivery, demotivate staff and usually fail in their objectives.

> Policy making has been rushed and is inadequately informed by understanding how the NHS ticks.

> The reforms are a recipe for disaster – a blend of a lack of insight, ineptitude and disregard for staff at all levels.
> (Walshe and Smith 2001: 21–3)

To summarise so far, although NHS managers may lack the vocational impulse which often is said to be the reason people choose to enter a profession, they are nevertheless influenced initially by the idea of doing worthwhile work for their fellow citizens in an organisation which, however vaguely defined, is said to represent public service values. As their experience expands, the tensions in endeavouring to satisfy the expectations of others may increase to a point where their original motivation is insufficient to keep them in the NHS. In such situations it is their expertise and managerial experience rather than claims to professionalism which is likely to obtain them another job.

Recently, top managers leaving the NHS have taken jobs at a national level in voluntary organisations, in academia and in quangos of various kinds. Only a minority enter the private sector, usually as management consultants. These mostly then work back in the public sector, suggesting that loyalty to public sector values is not entirely eroded by experience.

How others see NHS managers

The modernisation of the role of the health service manager, particularly since the introduction of general management, might have made managers feel better about their own standing. It did little, however, to recommend them to their clinical colleagues who saw managers drifting further away from a caring mode and from sorting out operational glitches.

The popular, lay view of health service managers is even less flattering. It is a continually reiterated complaint in the press and elsewhere that there are increasing numbers of managers in the system, consuming resources which would be better spent on direct patient care. It is in vain that managers or, occasionally, government ministers endeavour to put the facts of the case comparing management costs in the NHS favourably with those of other countries' health systems. Managers and their product, bureaucracy, are popularly considered to be unnecessary. It is strange that anyone faced with such a degree of general opprobrium would wish to do this sort of work. Possibly, managers perceive the popular scorn to be only skin-deep, largely symbolic, satisfying the public's need to find a scapegoat to accommodate adversity. Or perhaps managers' need to serve the common good overrides the lack of popular support.

Would professional status be advantageous?

Professional status might be considered desirable both by managers and by those they serve. With such status would come a statement of values, regulation of behaviour and, for the managers themselves, a sense of belonging which might protect them from constant criticism about their legitimacy.

Some degree of solidarity would appear to be necessary given the load now placed upon managers. There have recently been a number of scandals of malpractice within the NHS. Such issues are not new. Notoriously, management was held to account and found wanting in several hospitals for the elderly and people with mental illness and learning disabilities in the 1970s. However, because the cruelty those cases exposed was meted out largely by nurses, individual managers mostly escaped personal criticism and retribution. More recently, managers have been less able to evade personal accountability. They have even taken the blame for issues which previously would have been considered outside their remit, e.g. the clinical outcome of paediatric cardiac surgery (Bristol Royal Infirmary), the clinical practice of a gynaecologist (William Harvey Hospital, Ashford) or of a pathologist (Alder Hey Hospital, Liverpool).

The relationship of managers with government has become much more demanding. Notionally, it is the responsibility of whole NHS management boards to implement government policy. However, it is the executive health service managers who are charged with the actual task, whose importance, for the most senior managers, now appears to rank even higher than the more customary work of assuring patient welfare and ensuring financial control. The obligation to government is not new. What is different is the emphasis on the personal responsibility of individual key managers for achieving the government's aims.

There is a common perception that failure to give these aims explicit support leads to punishment. A survey of chief executives revealed 'Chief executives are expected to be cheerleaders for the reforms, not critics'. Furthermore, '... those chief executives who want to stay cannot afford to be seen as disloyal' (Walshe and Smith 2001: 23). This pressure has had deleterious effects on the organisations for which managers are responsible. Spurgeon and Barwell (2002: 24) note that many staff feel that they are not properly recognised for the work they do and that they have little influence on those decisions that impact on their work practices. This feeling is common across all staff groups except managers.

The publication of a *Code of Conduct for NHS Managers* (England only) (Department of Health 2002) could be seen as an attempt to reconcile some of the issues so far discussed.

This document first states the values which should underpin health service management for the guidance of managers themselves and those they serve. Secondly, it seeks to regulate managerial practice by stating what is required of managers. By attaching the Code to employment contracts, there is the intention (which may yet be contested as to its legal status) to make its requirements obligatory in line with the statutory requirements of clinical professionals. Thirdly, the Code aims to reassure the public that managers in the NHS will work to the highest standards. A fourth benefit might be seen to be that such a code, with its kinship to clinical professional codes, would enhance managers' status in the eyes of others and indeed their own.

Despite the possible advantages of the Code, its publication sharpens the fundamental issue as to whether managers can be seen as professionals, imitating their clinical colleagues, or whether it makes the situation even more confused than before.

What are NHS managers for?

Before coming to a conclusion as to the relevance or otherwise of professional status, it is worth exploring the basic question, what are managers for? Managers in the NHS have grown in importance. Some critics feel that they have become cuckoos in the nest. However, a kinder view would be that the complexity of the NHS has made it essential for there to be a group of people who are responsible for co-ordinating the often disparate aims of the organisation. Clinicians characteristically are concerned with the individual good of the patient in front of them. But it is clear that such a view has to be accommodated with a more general concern for the common good, for the whole organisation and its place in the national economy. The NHS Chief Executive's introduction to the Code acknowledges this:

> The interests of individual patients have to be balanced with the interests of groups of patients and of the community as a whole. The interests of patients and staff do not always coincide. Managerial and clinical imperatives do not always suggest the same priorities. A balance has to be maintained between national and local priorities.
>
> (Department of Health 2002: 1)

It is the manager's job, he implies, to endeavour to achieve this balance.

So why does this reasonable statement lead to difficulties? Criticism from clinicians is rooted in the managers' alleged lack of understanding of the needs of individual patients. Clinicians have habitually criticised managers for not representing their concerns about funding to the government. They have felt that managers are not 'on their side'. Managers, for their part, may well answer these criticisms by saying that it is their duty to manage what they have been given efficiently. To join clinicians in the demand for more would be to enter a political arena which, they feel, would compromise one aspect of their role as the implementers of government policy.

But has this function overtaken all others? The last ten years has seen the development of performance management with its plethora of outcome measures. League tables – currently a star-rating system – have assumed a disproportionate importance. Managers' work is now dominated by the need to reach government-determined targets. Those who fail, or who are seen as making false returns, are punished. This regime has damaging effects. The infantilising nature of a crude punishment and reward system has encouraged clinicians to see managers as immature, conformist and unsympathetic. This in turn increases the traditional antipathy between the two groups and thereby makes the management of the NHS much more difficult. Managers are seldom seen as allies and the co-operation of clinicians can only be bought by inducements.

If this rather pessimistic scenario has any validity, it must be asked why managers have allowed themselves to get into this position. Their occupational body, the Institute of Healthcare Management (IHM), is now over a century old. It claims to represent health service managers as a professional group. Despite various attempts to increase the number of members, only 10% of those who are involved in health service management belong to the IHM. It no longer sets examinations. Although it endeavours, through local and national events, to sponsor continuing education and development, its role is not sufficiently compelling for most managers to want to join. There is advantage in offering some critical evaluation of government policies from a corporate standpoint as this protects individual managers from political opprobrium. From time to time, largely determined by the personality and expertise of the current chief executive, the IHM has been the public voice of health service management regularly appearing in the media. However, this role has been inconsistently pursued.

It is clear that the IHM's desire to be recognised as a professional body is frail. Maybe it was always a misconceived ambition. Managers are, first and foremost, functionaries. Their role is to co-ordinate activity, to implement plans, to control resources. In a democracy, is it not reasonable that they should loyally implement the wishes of the government of the day? Paid from the public purse, is it not their duty to carry out instructions?

Certainly managers have an obligation to government, but that is not all. Even their code acknowledges a much more complex role:

- to make the care and safety of patients my first concern
- to respect the public, patients, relatives, carers, NHS staff and other agencies
- to show commitment to working as a team member
- to be honest and act with integrity.

(Department of Health 2002: 3)

Such statements of good intent are habitually found in codes of conduct. Unfortunately, the statements also contain contradictions. In this case, it is difficult to reconcile principles of honesty and integrity with what we might call the demands of politics. The code seeks to remove any ambiguity but in so doing increases the tension:

> For the avoidance of doubt, nothing [in the previous paragraphs] requires or authorises a NHS manager to whom their code applies; ... to make, permit or knowingly allow to be made any disclosure in breach of his or her duties and obligations to his or her employer, save as permitted by law.
>
> (Department of Health 2002: 5)

Such a stricture can be interpreted as a curb on the right of a NHS manager to criticise government policy, however constructively. In this respect, professional status would offer some protection.

So there are contrary arguments. On the one hand, NHS managers have few of the fundamental attributes attached to professions, such as control of entry and exit, self-regulation and an exclusive body of knowledge. On the other hand, because they are increasingly blamed by government for unsuccessful policies and by the public for the general inefficiencies of the system, some form of occupational solidarity would help managers to present a more realistic view of what is and is not possible in the running of the NHS, without being punished for so doing.

Public servants or civil servants?

Despite the protection afforded by corporate solidarity, it is my view that the debate on whether or not health service managers should seek to give themselves professional status leads to a conclusion that so doing is to misrepresent their essential role. Few feel the need to belong to a professional body, the IHM. More belong to a trade union. Significantly, the most senior have recently joined a union which principally represents senior civil servants. This may well be the nub of the issue. Are health service managers civil or public servants? Indeed, is there any point in drawing a distinction between the two?

The argument in favour of accepting civil servant status is that it removes some of the tensions that now exist. NHS managers' prime purpose would be to implement the policies of the elected government. Debates on the desirable level of resources and on the wisdom of policy changes are essentially political and would not therefore be the immediate concern of managers. Decisions about rationing patient care would be passed up the line to the government or its agencies, such as the National Institute for Clinical Excellence, to resolve. The prime purpose of managers would be to do what they are best at – getting things done. Such an action-oriented role has appeal for many managers whom, as we have seen, were originally attracted to the job by the level of responsibility and the variety of activity.

Nevertheless, the limitations of this fundamentalist approach are immediately apparent. First, it is unlikely to be effective. The evidence is that organisations seldom thrive under an essentially authoritarian regime governed by performance targets. Doctors over the years have demonstrated their ability to thwart governments' intentions. Increasing the sanctions which could be imposed by local management at the behest of central government would make matters worse and exacerbate the cultural divide which already damages doctor–manager relationships.

Secondly, using managers as merely the servants of government would be likely to kill innovation in the interests of loyalty to the government of the day. Twenty years ago, a study noted that the top managers at that time most valued the discretion that allowed them to balance local needs with national policies (Stewart *et al.* 1980). Today much of that choice has been lost under the weight of top-down directives. The *NHS Plan*'s 'earned autonomy' suggests that local initiatives can only be tolerated once national targets have been met. This effectively means that there will be little time for innovation despite the fact that new ideas are more likely to come from local practice than from central government.

Thirdly, public servants have an ethos based on service to local communities. They are more able to represent the consequences of intended policy change back to the government. However, increasingly they have been discouraged from doing this; any form of criticism, however constructive and well validated by experience, has been unwelcome. Consequently, the distinction between being a public servant and being a civil servant has become blurred.

Finally, managers cannot expect to provide effective leadership if they are perceived to be lackeys of some external power. Numerous studies have shown that where there are shared values within an organisation, it is easier to agree common purpose. Health service managers already have considerable difficulty in reconciling managerial imperatives with clinical aims. Creating further distance between the manager and the rest of the staff would lead to unhappy and dysfunctional organisations.

Conclusion

The ethic of the public servant might be defined as being an advocate of public needs, to act as a custodian of public assets and to be a steward of the common good. If health service managers are to fulfil this role they need to redefine their current position. Can they only do this through some appeal to professional status?

Such status might increase their sense of occupational solidarity. This in turn would strengthen their negotiating power with government. However, most managers are not persuaded of the need to do that. Because of this, their claims to professional status are always likely to be unconvincing.

It would be more helpful in promoting the common good if NHS managers, together with similar managers in other parts of the public sector, were to reconsider their obligations as public servants. They need to attempt to reduce the ambiguity of their role and recalibrate the balance between national policies and local needs. Currently NHS managers, working under greater pressure than before from a government committed to changing the management of the public sector, are too willing to accede to every top-down directive. In so doing, they are failing to represent the bottom-up views of the communities they should be serving. They are also undervaluing the wisdom they have accrued from years of experience in running health services. In this situation, seeking professional recognition is largely an irrelevance.

CHAPTER 6

Equity versus efficiency: managing competing values for the public sector leisure professional

Stephen Howell and Michael McNamee

Introduction

Most professionals work within a framework in which their organisations' overall aims, objectives and values are publicly stated. Traditionally understood, the private sector is driven characteristically by the overarching value of profit making whereby customers' desires provide commercial imperatives. By contrast, the public sector is driven by the value of service which responds to citizens' needs. Each sector, together with its constituent organisations and institutions, is shaped by the relevant values dominant in those spheres.

There are an increasing number of places in which the traditional absolute dichotomies between public and private sectors and their respective values have fallen away. Here, the values of profit and service mingle and often collide. The leisure services of local authorities are one such place.

Public leisure services operate within a pseudo-market created by local authorities. Here there are significant areas of overlap with the private sector. The non-statutory status of leisure provision often results in local authorities seeking to withdraw expenditure from these services in difficult financial times. This results in an operating environment in which issues of equity and efficiency collide on a regular basis. The role of mediating between these values often falls to leisure professionals. They find themselves caught up in a confusion of local and national policies and structures that undermine the very ground of professionalism.

This chapter provides an account of how leisure professionals have to manage, mediate, and resolve conflicting fundamental values within their work. It focuses on the clash between equity, a public service value, and efficiency, a private sector value. We will highlight conflicts such as those between equity and efficiency initially from a theoretical viewpoint, that of utilitarianism. This underlies much thinking in public policy and provision. Then we will move to look at the more concrete contextual and structural situations in which leisure professionals are required to undertake their necessary task of mediation between conflicting interests and values. We outline some ways in which leisure professionals might situate themselves in relation to political structures to mediate the conflict between equity and efficiency. We hope to demonstrate that leisure professionals as moral agents working in a particular context are constantly having to undertake value management as a fundamental, unavoidable part of their role.

Before advancing to look at managing the specific value conflict between equity and efficiency, it is important briefly to sketch out the assumptions that underlie our analysis. Thus we shall deal first with the fundamentally moral nature of professionalism and then describe the context in which leisure professionals operate, before proceeding to spell out our assumptions about the character and content of the provision of leisure services that frame our analysis of the values of equity and efficiency issues.

The moral nature of professionalism

Understandings of the essence of being a profession or professional are disputed. Bayles (1981) sets out three definitive criteria for professional status being accorded:

- extensive training
- intellectual training in kind
- training is related to an important service.

These criteria are very limited. They lack a qualitative aspect. Above all, they are inherently technical rather than moral. They do not recognise the moral ends, authority and responsibility invested in traditional professions by their members and by the public. Recognising a sense of moral purpose with its accompanying responsibility as central to professional identity and activity is essential to account for the trust that the public have in certain powerful occupational groups granted considerable authority over important spheres of human life.

It is our assumption here that one of the main distinguishing features of any occupational group that can appropriately be designated a profession is that it has moral ends, authority, responsibility and management invested in it. Its members are expected habitually to act with a degree of judgement, including value and moral judgement. All professionals need to mediate and manage values. It will be seen that this is certainly the case in the situation of contemporary leisure professionals. Unfortunately, a focus on everyday operational issues can easily obscure the more complex normative and value issues that tacitly undergird their daily work.

Public sector leisure services and professionals

For public local authorities, the provision of leisure services is an attempt to provide services that benefit local communities by improving the quality of life of their residents. This is achieved in a number of ways, for example by the provision of open space, sporting and arts facilities, or by ensuring access to other events and activities.

There is a variety of professional groups engaged in the provision of leisure services at different levels from national planners and policy makers through to individuals with particular skills (e.g. in sport or the arts) working with small groups of people at the neighbourhood level. Our concern in this chapter is mainly with professional leisure managers whom we regard here as the paradigmatic example of leisure professionals.

There are different levels of leisure management from senior leisure managers whose concerns are mainly with national and regional policy, planning and intervention, through middle managers whose roles revolve around community policy and planning, to those at local level who are responsible for day-to-day operations and systems of delivery. We take professional leisure managers at the first two levels as the paradigmatic example of the leisure professions here.

The context of public sector leisure provision and the normative demands of professionalism

Given the artificial scarcity of leisure, which is prescribed by budget rather than consumption, leisure professionals are consistently required to balance the legitimacy and feasibility of any pattern of allocation against a coherent perspective of the service.

A number of competing demands are made upon the professional in leisure, as in any other part of the public sector. Leisure professionals feel pressures from different stakeholders in many different quarters, e.g. from the general public, elected local authority members, central government and quangos like the Arts Council and Sport England. Their task would be unproblematic under conditions of consensus and coherence of interests. However, such harmony rarely exists. The leisure professional must therefore mediate between the conflicting values inherent in the social policy directives of central government, local community views and, quite often, local political views. These, characteristically, conflict and compete. Unclear, often contradictory, social policy frameworks only compound the situation.

Most leisure professionals currently work in an environment that attempts to promote open-ended political agendas through policy directives such as social inclusion, which serves the value of increasing equity. This aspiration must be worked towards within the constraints of increasing fiscal retrenchment for local authorities, which pushes services towards the values of economy, effectiveness and efficiency. Such conflict of values is not only in evidence between various policy directives. It can quite often be encompassed within a single view. The UK government policy of 'Best Value' is an exemplar to this confusion. We consider it briefly to demonstrate the lack of normative coherence that underpins it.

Value conflict: the example of the 'Best Value' policy

'Best Value' as a policy requires the leisure professional to comply with the following four C's:

- to *challenge* (outline the case for the leisure need at hand)
- to *compare* (with other authorities in order to benchmark their own provision and demonstrate effectiveness)
- to *consult* (with all stakeholders in order to determine the needs of the whole community)
- to *compete* (in order to ensure efficiency) so that they carry out their roles in a manner consonant with a profession that preserves their status and underwrites their responsibility with a professional ethic.

These directives present leisure professionals with a multitude of values for interpretation into service delivery plans. Conflicting values may appear to be a matter for strategic planners of leisure services. However, managers operating services must deal with them on a day-to-day basis. The process of implementing public sector policy poses deep philosophical problems that beset utilitarian thinking more generally (McNamee *et al.* 2000).

Analytic assumptions

We will make the following assumptions about leisure and leisure professionals in framing our analysis of the management of the value clash between equity and efficiency:

- leisure is a universal human need
- the state has a moral obligation to ensure that this need is met for all its citizens
- leisure should be understood as a certain class of activities and practices as opposed to a certain time slice (i.e. not work) (McNamee 1994)
- trust and authority are an integral part of the relationship between

leisure professionals and the public whose interests they are obliged to serve (McNamee *et al.* 2000).

The final assertion above implies that an important part of being a leisure professional, as with other traditional professional groups, is to assume moral authority and power in this sector.

A utilitarian approach to resolving value conflicts in leisure provision

The principle of utility is that actions shall be undertaken or policies adopted that have the end of promoting the greatest benefit of the greatest number of people. The attraction of utilitarian thinking in the public sector is that it apparently provides an impartial single framework through which dilemmas may be resolved. Within the public sector, the principle of utility requires that what should be sought is the greatest benefit to the most people in a way that caters for the needs and desires of those affected. To allow this to happen, what is needed is a system of accounting that informs professionals as to which options give best value. It is this that brings about the necessity for undertaking the cost–benefit analyses that have now become common in the public sector.

In the context of the present discussion two fundamental questions need to be answered here:

- Whose good matters most?
- Can we really compare and calculate leisure outcomes?

Unfortunately, fundamental questions like these are often glossed over in the apparent neutrality that cost–benefit analyses offer.

Whose good matters most?

Modern leisure services emerged from a paternalistic approach in which approved leisure activities were valued by providers principally because they promoted 'rational recreation' which would divert the masses from their licentious proclivities and bring them within the ambit of socially desirable, controlled behaviour. This paternalistic attitude, with its role for the leisure professional as an instrument of social control, has had its day. Newer, more democratic models of community practice and community development now emphasise the enabling and facilitating role of the professional (Butcher 1994: 3–25).

However, there are still unresolved and unconsidered issues about defining the outcomes and benefits of leisure activity. What knowledge and whose interests are to be used in defining the processes and the outcomes in this apparently democratic model? How are different interest groups to be involved? And who is to judge between the different ways of defining goods? How is this judgement to be undertaken?

A thoroughgoing utilitarian must be committed to educating, informing and identifying the desires of the relevant population under consideration rather than assuming such knowledge or being *inappropriately* swayed by minority or other interest groups. These theoretical criticisms bite hard on professional practice that seeks to be inclusive, equitable and accountable in practice as well as in theory.

Comparing and calculating leisure outcomes

A further problem for the utilitarian leisure professional urged to challenge and compare their strategies and methods of provision within the cost–benefit framework of 'Best Value', is that of aggregating individual benefits into some overall measure of social benefit. This presupposes comparability across goods. It also presupposes comparability across people. How can the leisure professional decide whether what one person has lost is more or less than another person has gained in consequence of a particular action? Utility refers essentially to private states of happiness or well-being. Taking a sophisticated, comprehensive and equitable measure of utility would require detailed knowledge of client preferences. This would commit leisure policy makers to massive data collection enterprises to gather the relevant information.

The limits of cost–benefit thinking in practice

The problems raised about utilitarian ways of thinking underlying the cost–benefit analysis approach to the provision of leisure services, together with the issues raised for the mediating professional worker, can be fleshed out more concretely by taking two examples, those of sports development services and the provision of new leisure facilities.

Sports development services

Sports development services are often seen as epitomising the drive by local authorities to ensure social justice or equity in leisure. The aims and objectives of all sports development schemes incorporate the need to provide the opportunity for all residents to participate in, or take up, sporting activities. Often, sports development schemes deliberately target those people within the community who are least likely to obtain those opportunities without some form of support or assistance. The current 'Active Communities' and

'Positive Futures' schemes, promoted by Sport England, are indicative of this kind of work.

In such a situation, the leisure professional seeks to attract more people to participate in sport *at the same time* as seeking to reach the target groups identified by social inclusion strategies. These are often groups who conspicuously fail to engage in a given range of leisure pursuits. However, if leisure professionals try to *maximise* participation levels, such groups would be unlikely to receive any attention. Indeed, where sports development becomes guided by values of efficiency, manifesting in a focus on income generation and participation levels, managers will react by seeking the line of least resistance. They would target existing participants to increase their levels of activity or encourage those groups already on the fringes of engagement and therefore relatively easy to contact. Such people might often be white, middle-aged males with relatively higher levels of disposable income – clearly not a category whose preferences were being prioritised by the original strategy.

Whose good matters? In philosophical parlance, this problem is known as the 'impossibility of interpersonal utility comparisons' (Goodin 1991: 241ff). (For a utilitarian objection to this standard criticism, *see* Brandt 1992.) It seems insurmountable. Having said this, however, a failure to make interpersonal utility comparisons could result in either completely random leisure provision or, ultimately, no leisure provision at all.

Providing leisure facilities

We may observe precisely the same kinds of difficulties in the allocation and distribution of leisure facilities. In considering any new leisure facility, a professional's role is to mediate and advise between conflicting interest groups to provide a range of appropriate sustainable services which match the needs of the community as closely as possible within the resources available.

In public policy this exemplifies the classic equity and efficiency dilemma (Lineberry 1977; Crompton and Wicks 1986, 1990; Coalter 1998; Hague *et al.* 2000). For example, there may be considerable community and local political support for the provision of a new swimming pool within a local authority. The argument put forward might rest on the self-evident health benefits that access to such a facility would bring to all the adults and children in the community. On the other hand, such provision will involve the authority in considerable expense and mean that other services and facilities will not be provided or expanded. Here, leisure professionals can play a major role by using their judgements to mediate between values of the community and those of corporate responsibility.

Such dilemmas do not always reduce to considerations of fairness. Often fiscal prudence and political expedience will prevail. Yet still the leisure professional ought always to consider whether it is fair to deny a community access to a swimming pool. Is it fair to provide a swimming pool at the cost of other services? This can be seen as a value conflict between equity and efficiency. It can also be regarded as a problem of redistribution. Leisure professionals must consider how such expenditure on leisure goods relates to other goods and services provided by the authority.

It is questionable how useful simplistic models of cost–benefit analysis are in situations of incommensurable goods and services. Cost–benefit analysis considers the marginal ability of an authority to find the necessary resources, resources which for the most part are unlikely to be available to provide the facility. Once leisure professionals pose the question 'what are the redistributional consequences of providing this facility?', they can mediate more effectively between the values of equity and efficiency. They may thus assist their local authorities in their decision making.

In such circumstances, the professional has the opportunity to legitimise their role. It is easy for local authorities and their officers to aspire to new, prestigious facilities to satisfy national agendas or local political pride. It is the proper role of the leisure professional here to provide guiding insight into whether the decision is feasible and efficient, but also to ensure that it embodies equity-driven values as well. In this context we advocate value-driven, responsible professionalism over the concerns of technical efficiency that form a façade for flawed and limited cost–benefit analysis based on superficial utilitarian thinking.

Leisure professionalism: structures and decision making

Reflective awareness of value conflicts is a precondition of professionalism in any robust sense of the word. The responsible leisure professional must be aware that the equity and efficiency conflict is not just a personal problem or a battle of ideas. It is also a social issue requiring consideration and mediation of the interests of a wide range of stakeholders.

An awareness and understanding of the procedures that can procure greater equity at a local level must assist the leisure professional's role in determining how resources are to be allocated. The just allocation of services and goods should be based not only on the internal logic and values of the good at hand, i.e. leisure services, but also on an appreciation of local citizens' understandings of the good life, its values and activities (*see* Howell and McNamee 2003).

Having positioned the leisure professional as the mediator of conflicting values, they are faced with two major influences on their ability to discharge this responsibility. The first of these is the *organisational structure for decision making*, in particular the prevailing political structure. The second is the *mechanism of service delivery* employed by the authority. These parameters are likely to determine the role and scope of the leisure professional's position within the organisation. They will influence his or her ability to mediate competing values.

The committee system of local authorities

In relation to political structure, the committee systems found within most local authorities provide a very good example. Because they are representative of specific service interests or groups of services (i.e. community services, financial services), local authority committees usually make decisions about single value issues.

For example, a community or leisure-based committee examining play services will characteristically focus fairly narrowly on the level, nature and scope of this specific provision. It is unlikely to give any serious consideration to how any action it recommends is related to the authority's wider plans. Questions of how such services will directly link to the revenue, capital or the corporate aspirations of the local authority will probably be ignored.

Politicians, who also face conflicting demands for equity and efficiency from the electorate, are able to champion different values at different committees without any obvious contradiction in their position. The same politician can support values of equity through, for example, a leisure committee and values of efficiency through financial committees. The result of this separation of discussion of values by time and space is that appropriate rhetoric can be produced and open conflict among the politicians reduced. However, the dilemmas and the conflict still remain for the officials, such as the leisure professionals. They have to advise their councillors and implement the decisions.

Service delivery mechanisms

The delivery mechanism has a significant role to play in shaping the leisure professional's ability to mediate on the conflicting values of equity and efficiency. An important role for leisure professionals working for local authorities in the recent past has been that of acting as client officer. A client officer is the local authority official with responsibility for overseeing that a council's interests are fulfilled by a third party acting on the authority's behalf, e.g. a supplier of leisure services. These interests are normally clearly expressed within a service level agreement or contract specification. Often, client officers were the senior leisure professionals within a local authority. They had considerable responsibility and scope for mediating values and determining the nature and delivery of services in line with the outcomes of value deliberation as outlined above.

The professional role of client officer is now threatened with extinction and/or reduction in scope because, increasingly, different kinds of organisations and charitable leisure trusts are being used as delivery agents. A delivery agent is the organisation with responsibility for delivering a service. In addition to charitable trusts, other public bodies such as parish councils, voluntary sector organisations and the private sector may be engaged by a local authority. These delivery agents have increasing autonomy as time goes on.

The proliferation of these different agents of service delivery may result in a general decline in claims to professionalism by leisure professionals. There may be an erosion of most senior-based leisure posts within local authorities matched by an increased claim to professional status from delivery agents, as the role and scope of such agents expand. However, as the autonomy and responsibilities of these agents grow, they will need to have regard to the issues of equity and effectiveness presently mediated by local authority-employed leisure professionals. Trusts and agents of various kinds should in fact be capable of mediating responsibly between conflicting values and competing interest groups. To do so, however, they must be invested with the ability to act paternalistically in autonomy-respectful ways to fulfil people's leisure needs. To facilitate this, local authorities will have to accept a certain loss of control over services and be more willing to trust the organisations they engage to deliver services for them. Moreover, such new organisations must escape from the mentality of competitive tendering. They need to rationalise the delivery of leisure services not as a simple financial transaction with the authority, but with commitment to the role of leisure in people's lives in a more thoroughgoing, value-sensitive manner.

Conclusion

The nature, role and scope of public sector leisure provision will continue to change. This will affect the roles and responsibilities of leisure professionals within local authority settings. One thing will not change. There will continue to be a need to mediate effectively between the increasingly conflicting values of efficiency and equity. This ongoing need may appear to strengthen the case for having leisure professionals who situate their role within the understanding of a professional as moral agent who is responsive and responsible in mediating and managing fundamental values through a process of skilled judgement.

The task of mediating and managing values is a complex and demanding one which should not be underestimated. The temptation may be to opt out of this kind of professional work and to resolve complex tensions and conflicts by ignoring one set of issues – pursuing efficiency without regard to equity or vice versa. We hope we have shown here that the losses involved in this kind of professional dereliction would be considerable and socially and individually damaging. Thus, whatever the problems in theory and practice bound up with performing effectively as a leisure professional in the public sector, this professional calling must be upheld as a practical ideal in some form. There will continue to be a fundamental need for professional mediators and managers of values in the public sector until such time as the state no longer sees itself as having a role in meeting the leisure needs of all its citizens.

The ability of leisure managers to bring solutions to the equity versus efficiency dilemma puts an onus on them to trade effectively in values. Whether such managers are situated within local authority leisure departments, direct service organisations or charitable trusts, they require moral authority in order to be effective and equitable. It is only by investing leisure managers with moral authority and by attending to non-technical aspects of their professional socialisation that we can hope to resolve the many day-to-day operational issues highlighted here.

CHAPTER 7

Value dilemmas and social work practice

Jeremy Roche

Introduction

I want to argue here that while values are central to contemporary social work education and practice, their realisation is a complex matter. The language of values is fundamental to social work's definition of itself. However, the clarity of professional value statements and the relationship between values and practice is problematic. This is not simply a consequence of particular dilemmas which are inherent to social work.

To set the scene for this discussion, I review the regulatory framework governing social work before going on to consider the distinct but interconnected sources of 'values talk' which impact on social work practice. I then examine how social work's value commitment can be realised on a daily basis as well as the obstacles to such realisation. These obstacles are considerable. Without intending to set up an opposition between values and the rules that theoretically govern practice, arguably it is the commitment of individual professional social workers to ethical practice, rather than organisational compliance, which secures good practice and the interests of service users.

The regulatory framework

The regulatory framework governing social work is complex. It includes law, guidance and statutory regulations as well as professional codes of practice. For example, local authority social workers working in the field of child protection not only have to know about their powers and duties under the Children Act 1989, they also need to know about government guidance which provides further 'advice' as to how to conduct a child protection investigation. The professional social worker is also an employee and is bound by agency policies and procedures. Of course, on paper these policies and procedures should be in turn consistent with the overarching legal framework.

Law and the social worker today

The law spells out the powers and duties that social work has in a range of situations. It accords wide-ranging discretionary powers to intervene and regulate family life, e.g. to protect children. The law provides the authority upon which professional social work activity takes place and within which professional discretion is exercised. In the past, however, knowledge of the law was not seen as integral to good social work education and practice.

In the 1980s and 1990s, the law acquired an ever-increasing importance within social work (*see* generally Vernon *et al.* 1990). This was partly due to a series of scandals about the ways in which local authorities discharged their social service functions. Two of these illustrate one of the key dilemmas facing social work professionals, namely whether and how to intervene in family life.

In the Jasmine Beckford case, the local authority social services department failed to take action to prevent her death at the hands of her parents. The inquiry into her death found, amongst other things, much confusion about what could and could not be done under the law and that the social workers involved treated the parents as the client rather than the child (Blom Cooper 1985: 294). The media response to this event was one of condemnation of the social workers involved for their failure to take timely action to protect the child.

The inquiry into the Cleveland scandal, by contrast, criticised a range of professionals (including paediatricians, police and social workers) for their overzealous approach to protecting the children they believed to be at risk of sexual abuse. Here the main 'villains' were consultant paediatricians not social workers. In the words of the inquiry report:

> By reaching a firm conclusion on the basis of physical signs and acting as they would for non-accidental injury or physical abuse; by separating children from their parents and by admitting most of the children to hospital, [Dr Higgs and Dr Wyatt] compromised the work of the social workers and the police.
>
> (Butler-Sloss 1988: 243)

Nonetheless, the situation in Cleveland was seen as an instance of the local authority overreaching itself, even though it took the actions it did on the basis of the diagnoses of two doctors. For some children the child protection process itself was experienced as abusive – as the report observed, 'the voices of the children were not heard' (Butler-Sloss: 25). One of the messages from these inquiries 'read' by social workers was that they were damned if they did (intervene) and damned if they didn't.

The outcomes of these inquiries included reform of the law and a new emphasis on the fact that social work operated within a statutory framework. The Children Act 1989 redrew the relationship between the local authority, the courts and the family. There was an emphasis on working in partnership with families and children in need, and on clearer powers and duties of local authorities, with new procedural rights for parents.

The impact of human rights legislation

Today the law has a more central role in the world of social work. It is also clear that the law itself enshrines (however imperfectly) certain key values. These include, at least at the formal level, a commitment to equality of treatment, procedural fairness and respect for individual rights. With the coming into force of the Human Rights Act 1998, it is arguable that this aspect of the law has assumed a greater significance.

Article 1 of the European Convention on Human Rights (ECHR) states that the parties to the ECHR must 'secure to everyone within their jurisdiction the rights and freedoms' contained in the Convention. The UK Human Rights Act (HRA) 1998 incorporated most of the provisions of the ECHR into domestic law. Consequently, UK courts and tribunals are required to interpret and give effect to the law in a way which is compatible with the Convention rights (section 3 HRA 1998). The HRA also provides that it is unlawful for a public authority, which includes local authority social services departments, to act in a way which is incompatible with a Convention right (section 6 HRA 1998). The effect of the HRA 1998 is to make it easier to raise directly claims that one's human rights have been breached; professionals and service users alike come within the protections of the ECHR.

The regulatory bodies

Alongside this fluid legal structure there exists a rapidly changing professional scene. Throughout the UK regulatory bodies for social work have been established. These institutions, e.g. the General Social Care Council in England and the Scottish Social Services Council, are similar to those that operate for medicine, the law and nursing. They took up responsibility for the regulation of social work in 2001. There is, therefore, a multiplicity of regulations, advice and guidance on values and practice available to the social worker.

Registration with the regulatory councils is a condition of employment in the personal social services. The register's primary function is to protect the public and to set standards for those groups working in the social services field. In part, these new regulatory institutions arose out of ongoing public concern over examples of serious misconduct and bad practice by a minority of those working in the personal social services.

Over a million people work in the personal social services, providing social work and social care for very large numbers of children and adults who are often physically, emotionally and socially vulnerable. The regulatory councils have statutory powers to define and enforce standards and to investigate complaints and impose sanctions. These may include suspension, or exclusion, from the register.

The councils have published codes of practice and guidance material. This allows service users to know what they can expect, and practitioners and their employers to have a common understanding of conduct and practice requirements. In England, the General Social Care Council's Code of Practice (2002) states that social care workers must:

- protect the rights and promote the interests of service users and carers
- strive to establish and maintain the trust and confidence of service users and carers
- promote the independence of service users while protecting them as far as possible from danger or harm
- respect the rights of service users while seeking to ensure that their behaviour does not harm themselves or other people
- uphold public trust and confidence in social care services
- be accountable for their practice and take responsibility for maintaining and improving their knowledge and skills.

Thus there is a very clear commitment to value-based or ethical practice.

Professional codes: past and present

However, earlier social work texts also evinced a similar commitment to ethical practice. For example, in the Central Council for the Education and Training in Social Work (CCETSW) Revised Rules and Requirements (1995), the section on 'Values of Social Work' made it clear that meeting the core competencies central to good social work practice could only be achieved through the satisfaction of the 'value requirements'. The position was that 'values are integral to, rather than separate from competent practice' (CCETSW 1995: 18) and 'practice must be founded on, informed by and capable of being judged against a clear value base'.

These values requirements included the demands that students should 'identify and question their own values and prejudices and their implications for practice' and promote 'people's rights to choice, privacy, confidentiality and protection, while recognising and addressing the complexities of competing rights and demands' (CCETSW 1995: 18).

The current Code of Practice for Social Service Workers resembles the CCETSW rules and requirements. The language is at times different, however, a positive respect for the rights and interests of service users is common to both documents, as is the promotion of the independence of service users whilst ensuring they are protected. The Code of Practice also emphasises the issue of public trust and confidence in social services.

More recently, the Scottish Executive has observed (2003: 18):

> Social work has always had a strong ethical basis that emphasises the importance of building a positive, professional relationship with people who use services as well as with professional colleagues.... They must be able to understand the implications of, and to work effectively and sensitively with, people whose cultures, beliefs or life experiences are different from their own. In all of these situations, they must recognise and put aside any personal prejudices they may have, and work within guiding ethical principles and accepted codes of professional conduct.

In a similar vein, the British Association of Social Workers (BASW), in its Code of Ethics, adopted a definition of social work from the International Federation of Social Workers. This views the social work profession as promoting 'social change, problem solving in human relationships and the empowerment and liberation of people to enhance well-being' (BASW 2001). The Code of Ethics emphasises that social work is committed to five basic values:

- human dignity and worth
- social justice
- service to humanity
- integrity
- competence.

The standards for social work practice

Finally, the National Occupational Standards (hereafter referred to as the Standards) also position values and ethics as central to competent social work practice. In each of the 21 units contained in the Standards, values and ethics are separately considered. In demonstrating competence against these Standards, account must be taken of the Code of Practice.

There can be no doubt that a competent contemporary social work professional is required to be committed to ethical practice and to act accordingly. Their practice should be informed by respect for diversity and for the individual person, openness of communication, and a determination to counter discrimination and disadvantage.

The two important questions we must then pose are how is this commitment translated into practice in everyday professional life? And, what obstacles are there to the realisation of this commitment?

The significance of values

There has been considerable debate over values within social work literature. Braye and Preston-Shoot (1998) see the value base as central to social
work, but they also see its definition as open. It might refer to 'a commitment to respect for persons, equal opportunity and meeting needs' or more
radically to a 'concern with social rights, equality and citizenship' (1998:
59). They are not the only commentators who have identified an uncertainty in the meaning of social work's value base. Banks writes that most
decisions in social work involve a complex interaction of ethical, political,
technical and legal issues, but then goes on to observe that 'values' is 'one
those words that tends to be used rather vaguely and has a variety of
different meanings' (Banks 1995: 4).

Shardlow takes the argument further:

> Getting to grips with social work values and ethics is rather like
> picking up a live, large and very wet fish out of a running stream.
> Even if you are lucky enough to grab a fish, the chances are that
> just when you think you have caught it, the fish will vigorously
> slither out of your hands and jump back in the stream. . . . Values
> and ethics similarly slither through our fingers for a variety of
> reasons.
>
> (Shardlow 1998: 30)

It is not just a question of the openness or vagueness of the word 'values';
he argues that 'no consensus exists about value questions in social work'
(Shardlow 1998: 23). Shardlow refers to debates within social work over
whether the contract culture empowers clients, the extent to which social
work is predicated on a respect for the individual person, the significance of
ideology in social work (for example, the impact of feminism on social work
knowledge and practice in the 1980s and 1990s) and the extent to which
social workers should be held responsible when something goes wrong:

> These debates are inevitably open-ended where social work itself is
> intrinsically political, controversial and contested, and where the
> nature of practice is subject to constant change.
>
> (Shardlow 1998: 24)

Ambiguities surrounding social work encounters

Clark picks up on this theme when he observes that while everyone is agreed
that professionals are 'distinguished by their special knowledge and expertise', the actual task in which social workers are engaged centres on 'the
preoccupations of ordinary life'; 'the primary knowledge of social workers lies
within the realms of everyday know-how and life experience' (Clark 2000:

85–6). This ambiguity of social work expertise generates many awkward issues, for instance the comparative ease with which social work interventions can be challenged, as contrasted with those of medicine and law.

'Ordinary people' naturally have views about social work practice. They have opinions on issues such as the balance to be struck between the public interest in protecting the vulnerable and family privacy, the basis upon which interventions are made, and the potentially coercive aspect of social work. Precisely because they *do* have views, social work practice is never free of controversy, even when there are no recurring scandals besetting the profession. Social workers acting as advocates, or as gateways to much-needed resources, play a different role, are perceived differently, and have different effects on their clients' lives compared with when they act as organisers of coercive intervention and gatekeepers of scarce resources.

Indeed, while mostly engagements with professionals in general are characterised by choice where the clients *choose* to engage their services, this is often not the case when encountering a social worker. Service users are often driven to seek support from social services or are the unwilling objects of the gaze of social work. Some make use of social work services, while others have these 'services' thrust upon them.

In this context, the inequality of power characteristic of the service user–social worker relationship assumes a particular importance. If the service user is a reluctant participant in the social work process, then the social work ideals of empowering service users, promoting their participation and working in partnership with them are critical; how else is the social worker even to begin to realise the professional commitment to protect the rights and promote the interests of service users?

'Clients' or 'service users'?

Smith (1997) argues that the application of values is not without difficulty but goes on to note that a change in 'values talk' has taken place. For example, there has been a change in vocabulary towards referring to 'service users' rather than 'clients'. Perhaps this signals, among other things, a recognition of the proper agency of the vulnerable who need and use social work services.

It is axiomatic within social work that working in partnership with service users, empowering them and, if required, advocating on their behalf are core competencies. The idea that the vulnerable might have some insight, and therefore some cognitive authority over their own situation, is central to the theory of social work practice.

Here the question of rights becomes important. The idea of, and language of, rights is linked to what Smith designates 'fundamental human need'. Smith sees values and rights as conceptually distinct. However, she also sees in the idea of fundamental human need, itself predicated upon respect for the person, a positive link in the values–rights relationship.

That said, Smith raises some questions about the real significance of the language of rights within social welfare provision. Smith's concern is that 'rights are in danger of becoming dislocated from values' in a way that means values become invisible. So while the social work professional can be seen as a legal agent, this is not to say that the law totally defines and circumscribes practice; as Clark argues, 'social workers are rightly devoted to realising a wider conception of welfare' (Clark 2000: 110). In other words, the legitimacy of social work extends beyond law's reach.

Social work values: from theory to practice

Whatever the significance of shifts in language, respect for persons and self-determination remain central to social work practice. The complexity of the social work task relates in part to how the professional social worker negotiates the tension between social work values and the decision-making dilemmas that are integral to social work. However, it is axiomatic within social work scholarship that values do not only underpin social work practice and decision making. They also structure social work knowledge and research and thus feed into assessment of needs and interventions.

If assessment, the need for intervention and the nature of intervention are themselves a matter of subjective, albeit professional, judgement, then what is it that structures this judgement? Is it the personal values of the professional or professional values? The uncertainty which is central to social work practice – an uncertainty which can relate to the nature of the problem at issue as well as how to respond – requires the professional to be as clear as they can about the evidential basis on which they are contemplating taking action.

One of the recommendations of the Laming Report (2003) into the death of eight-year-old Victoria Climbie is that 'the Department of Health should amalgamate the current *Working Together* (1999) and the National Assessment Framework documents into one simplified document'. This proposal was aimed at achieving:

- a common language for use across agencies
- dissemination of best practice
- prescription of 'a clear step-by-step guide on how to manage a case ... with built-in systems for monitoring and review' (Laming Report 2003: 366).

The existence of such a guide might be seen as undermining of the very idea of professional judgement – a highly trained and experienced individual coming to a view as to what action, if any, to take.

In his analysis of risk and professional judgement, Parton argues that, with the increasing emphasis on accountability and the increase in ever more prescriptive regulations and guidance, the welfare practitioner is at risk of being reduced to an organisational functionary (Parton 2001: 62). An illustration of this is provided by the Framework for the Assessment of Children in Need and their Families. This outlines the process and the time limits within which assessment of children in need and parenting capacity should be analysed (Department of Health 2000a: 33). However, it could be argued that such a guide is simply an aid to professional judgement, not a substitute. It provides a distillation of best practice with a valuable framework for critical action and decision-making points.

As well as using guides, social work values can also be realised through an emphasis on evidence-based practice. Evidence-based practice informs social work professionals what works and it is argued that 'what works' is also practice which is value-based. For example, working in partnership is supportive of protecting the rights and promoting the interests of service users and carers and has been shown by research to produce better results; not only are the outcomes improved, but so are relations with service users (Department of Health 1995). Perhaps, at a deep level, social work values are to be realised through the securing of a sense of ownership for them in the workplace. This could be done by practitioners avoiding being judgemental themselves and challenging inappropriate behaviour and disrespectful speech directed towards service users and colleagues.

Obstacles to value-based practice

There are many quite powerful obstacles to value-based practice, not least of which is the failure to keep values central. At times this might certainly be hard to do. I have already mentioned briefly the contrast between Beckford and Cleveland. More recently, in contrast to the horrors of the Climbie case, there has been a different tragedy unfolding in the case of *P, C and S vs. United Kingdom* [2002] 2 FLR 631.

Victoria Climbie died at the hands of her great aunt and her partner. They were subsequently convicted of her murder. Over a period of 11 months, Victoria had had contact with three housing authorities, four social services departments, two child protection teams of the Metropolitan Police Service, the NSPCC and two hospitals. For the last four months of her life Victoria had no contact with social services. When she was admitted to hospital the day before she died, 'She was bruised, deformed and malnourished. Her temperature was so low it could not be recorded' (Laming Report 2003: 1). The cause of death was lung, heart and kidney failure. Dr Carey told the subsequent inquiry that 'In terms of the nature and extent of the injury and the almost systematic nature of the inflicted injury, I certainly regard this as the worst I have ever dealt with'. The Laming Report saw Victoria's death as due to the gross failure of the child protection system. The failings of professional judgement by front-line staff were compounded by the failure of management. In a final grotesque irony, on the day Victoria died, Haringey social services department had closed her file.

By contrast, in the case of *P, C and S*, the mother (*P*), a US citizen, had been married before and had had two children in that relationship. During 1994, the mother brought one of her two children to hospital on a number of occasions with complaints of fever and diarrhoea. It was discovered that the child had been given a laxative. The mother was prosecuted, convicted and put on probation. *C* was in the US doing research for his PhD on Munchausen's Syndrome by Proxy (MSP) when he met *P*, and in 1996 she left the US for the UK and married *C* in 1997. When she became pregnant by *C*, her former husband made the local authority aware of *P*'s previous history and conviction; neither *P* nor *C* accepted the label of MSP.

A pre-birth child protection case conference was then convened and the decision was taken to place the unborn child's name on the child protection register. The local authority also decided to apply for an emergency protection order (EPO) on the birth of the child rather than an interim care order as the latter would require the parents being given notice of the proceedings. The baby was removed from her mother on the day of her birth and subsequently only had supervised contact with her mother. The local authority then instituted care proceedings with adoption as part of the care plan: eventually the child was adopted.

There were a number of procedural irregularities which concerned the ECHR. However, on the matter of the application for an EPO *ex parte* in relation to the baby girl on birth, the ECHR decided that the EPO in itself was not contrary to article 8 of the ECHR, but the way in which it was implemented, i.e. the baby's removal, did breach article 8. The Court held that there must be extraordinarily compelling reasons before a baby can be physically removed from its mother against her will immediately after birth as a consequence of a procedure in which neither she nor her partner has been involved.

Social work practice in this case appears to fly in the face of the social work commitment to working in partnership with parents. It also breaches the parents' human rights. This appears to violate many of the principles and values that social workers claim to hold dear. The impression left is that of precipitate action with no effective redress available to the affected parties. By contrast, Climbie's case captures a failure to act and to supervise properly – which again represents a failure of social work values and ethics.

Perhaps the 'politics of risk' are part of the dilemma facing social work professionals. For a profession under siege, it might be difficult to avoid substituting the language of risk for that of need. It can be difficult to avoid reacting to the media attacks on the profession in any way other than 'playing it safe'. Unfortunately, in the context of working with children and families, playing it safe can too easily translate into simply removing the child.

The impact of professional hierarchies

It is important also to be honest about the impact of professional hierarchies on social workers. In the Cleveland scandal, Butler-Sloss (1988) referred to the social workers being misled by the paediatricians. In the Climbie case, Lord Laming argued that Dr Schwartz's diagnosis that Victoria was suffering from scabies should have been challenged (Laming Report 2003: 302). This diagnosis was made at one of the key moments in Victoria Climbie's life in the UK. She was taken to the Central Middlesex Hospital by her ex-child-minder and the duty doctor and the paediatric registrar had already formed suspicions that some of the child's injuries might be non-accidental. Victoria was placed under police protection and the medical notes recorded there were to be no unsupervised visits by her aunt (referred to as her mother in these notes). Dr Schwartz's scabies diagnosis resulted in the police protection coming to an end and Victoria being taken home the next morning.

But how is the social work professional to challenge the doctor? The professional 'pecking order' is such that only the most confident social worker who is sure of their ground will be able to challenge a member of the medical profession.

The Laming Report also severely criticised the poor management and supervision of the front-line social workers. It observed that senior management failed in their duty to their staff by not providing proper supervisory support. Indeed, the 'greatest failure' rested with the managers as opposed to the 'hapless if sometimes inexperienced' staff. For Lord Laming, among the many changes required was 'the drawing of a clear line of accountability, from top to bottom, without doubt or ambiguity about who is responsible at every level for the well-being of vulnerable children' (Laming Report 2003: 5).

While unsettling and uncomfortable for the social work professionals involved, social work practice must be called to account if the rhetoric surrounding respect for the individual and diversity is to have any meaning. If social work professionals routinely fail to listen to and work with service users (including children) and, among other things, respect their self-defined needs, then it is hard to see how their practice would not fall short of their professional commitment to 'values and ethics'.

Conclusion

Although this chapter could be interpreted as being highly critical of social work professionals, this is not my intention, despite the exploration of a number of obvious awkward issues facing them. At this stage, therefore, it is important to state two truths about social work:

● it is a highly complex task, requiring great skill and judgement if mistakes are to be avoided and vulnerable people are to be supported in solving the difficult problems they face

- it is also the case that social work practice is fundamentally about professional judgement, and very often that practice is executed with appropriate skill and decisiveness.

CCETSW argued that social workers had to

> ... recognise the interrelationships of structural and individual factors in the social context in which services operate, and the need to address their impact on the lives of children and adults.
>
> (CCETSW 1995: 18)

The problems that bring 'service users' and social workers together can be caused by the personal characteristics of service users. They can also be engendered by the pattern of disadvantages and inequalities that are built into the structure of our society. Indeed, those personal characteristics are affected by social inequalities. Therefore, in working with service users, social workers inevitably have to engage with the impact of these disadvantages and inequalities and decisions have to be made about the appropriate course of action.

However, the same set of facts can give rise to very different decisions. In work on the Children Act 1989, I found that different groups of social work professionals responded in radically different ways to the same practice scenarios. How is this to be explained? Part of the explanation is that the personal values (as opposed to the professional values) of the social work professional intrude. Moreover, different workplaces have different organisational cultures which impact on professional decision making. It is thus relevant to consider the induction of social work professionals into their workplace.

Perhaps this process, which runs alongside the more formal and statutory-based understandings of the obligations of the professional, is critical. All institutions in different ways induct new employees. It might be that the 'real story' of what it is like being a social worker 'here' and how to handle the practice dilemmas integral to practice is conveyed not via the formal rules but via the stories that arrivals are told about the workplace. Workplace practices and commitments might reinforce or undermine the formal messages of the law, codes of practice and the professionals' contracts of employment.

Ultimately, social work, like much complex professional activity, is not about rule following but is about professional judgement. Rules have their limits (Gould 1996). We noted earlier that, in social work, professional judgement is framed by the legal framework, agency policies and procedures, the individual social worker's contract with their employer, their professional knowledge and experience and their professional value base. Payne argues that social workers are required to do more than follow procedures, conventions or manuals. They have to think things through, apply lessons from past experience and find new ways to deal with new situations.

He, therefore, stresses the need for:

> ... maintaining a critical awareness that at any time we may need to think again and think differently. Because this kind of flexibility is the essence of dealing with any human being and being effective in working on complex human problems, critical awareness and reflection is [sic] an important practical implementation of the social work value of respecting human individuality and rights.
>
> (Payne 2002: 122)

In addition, however, while it is also framed by the social work professional's commitment to 'values and ethics', this commitment has to be placed in context. Too easily the rhetoric of concern about human rights and social justice can give way in individual cases to a disregard and erosion of the rights of service users. Languages of partnership, empowerment and anti-oppressive practice have to be operationalised in a context of severe resource constraints, genuine professional concern for the safety and well-being of other service users (if not themselves), and the reality of the ambiguous and uncertain situations that are characteristic of social work.

A commitment to value-based practice might result in social workers 'blowing the whistle' on their agency or colleagues. The following example illustrates how the organisational and managerial context of social work can undermine social work values:

> Social workers attending law workshops have recounted experiences of being instructed not to inform service users of their rights, and of users being charged for services which fall outside the legal mandate to charge.
>
> (Braye and Preston-Shoot 1998: 58)

Thus part of the social work task requires having the skills and professional commitment to challenge unfairness or illegality. Value-based practice presupposes a respect for service users and their rights and a professional commitment to act in support of the service user.

PART III

Values embodied in codes of practice

Introduction

One obvious focus for exploring the relationship between values and professional practice is in professional codes. If one wants to know exactly what a profession's view of itself and its values are, perhaps the first place to look should be in its own written code where, one might hope, its values will be set out clearly and unambiguously.

Most, but not all, professions have a code of ethics, conduct or practice which directly or indirectly outlines important values for professional members and gives guidance on how these values should be realised in practice. Indeed, it could be argued that it is one of the marks of an occupation claiming professional status that it should have such a code. Certainly, most of the professions discussed in this book (apart from the artistic profession) have issued guidance of one sort or another, if not formal codes.

The chapters in this part of the book centre on a number of different written professional codes with a view to examining what they might reveal – or not reveal – about the explicit and implicit values of professional groups. Despite their formal status and prominence in professional life, there are substantial complications and limitations in their practical use and implementation. Many professionals are aware of the existence of codes of practice but neglect their detailed contents in everyday life and work. Codes often prescribe ideals. Both members of professional groups and outsiders frequently witness these ideals being violated or negated in practice, not least because sometimes values and ideals clash with each other. Thus, there is a gap between the theoretical and the practical in relation to codes. This gap can sometimes be very wide indeed, raising questions about the real benefits of having a code at all. Why bother with codes, and why devote a section of the book to them?

Codes are important and deserve attention because their infringement can, in some cases, lead to suspension or expulsion from the profession. This has serious implications for an individual professional's status and income. Codes also reveal a great deal about a profession's formal working ideology and the way it wishes to be perceived externally. The use and neglect of the stipulations of codes by practitioners also throw considerable light upon the relationship between values and professional practice.

It would be possible simply to give a straight descriptive account of a representative selection of codes, their origin, composition and use. Here, however, these documents are considered in an evaluative way. As with anything to do with values, critical examination of codes raises some very interesting general issues about the interaction between values and practice. This interaction turns out to be rather more complicated than anticipated. Rather than simply taking codes at 'face value', it is necessary to dig deeper and recognise that such documents are products of a particular place and time; they should be understood in their context. They can be 'interrogated' by asking questions such as:

- for whom was this written?
- why was it written?
- when was it written?
- who wrote it?
- whose values does it embody?
- how is it, and how has it been, used?
- has it been revised? When and why?

Readers belonging to professional groups might be interested in putting these questions to their own professional codes.

In Chapter 8 'What can we expect of professional codes of conduct, practice and ethics?', Paul Wainwright, an academic nurse teacher and ethicist, and Stephen Pattison, a practical theologian with a background in health research and management, suggest that it is necessary to rethink conventional attitudes to the function and structure of codes. They do this by drawing an analogy with attitudes towards religious texts. Both codes and scriptural texts are often presented and read as unchanging, unquestionably valid, and uncontroversial. However, these texts require continuing dynamic interpretation in practice if they are to have an active, living importance.

Wainwright and Pattison suggest that, paradoxically, people expect both too much and too little from codes. Mainly using codes from the health sector to illustrate their argument, the authors show how codes are rarely very helpful in daily life – at least to those seeking an easy-to-apply set of rules which can be followed without too much thought. They also demonstrate that while codes are often very strong on rhetoric and the affirmation of high moral ideals, these ideals or values can also often be quite contradictory. Moreover, it is often not at all clear exactly whose interests are being served by the production of codes.

Wainwright and Pattison go on to argue that codes, as written texts, are of little use by themselves. They have to be interpreted. This is not a straightforward process. Furthermore, interpretations, like those of authoritative religious texts, will vary according to the person and the situation. The authors propose that instead of regarding professional codes as complete, unchangeable documents 'given from on high', it would be far better to think of them as dynamic and provisional working drafts to be challenged and debated far more openly. This might allow professionals to use their codes as a resource for aiding reflection about their daily work and developing reflective practice.

After Wainwright and Pattison's very critical, general and analytic piece, a fascinating, contrasting chapter which is much more specific and normative in its approach to codes is provided by James Armstrong. Armstrong is a civil engineer of considerable experience who has taken a very active part in the professional organisations of engineers throughout his working life. Armstrong's own interest in professional issues of values and ethics was based in his own experiences, particularly of overseas projects. In Chaper 9

'The development and use of codes for professional engineers', he gives an 'insider' account of his understanding of the role of the codes in practice for his profession and describes the background and development of the code of practice to which he personally contributed.

Armstrong is in no doubt about the importance of this normative code, or of the need for it. Indeed, he believes that every professional group needs one as part of its guidance to members. His growing awareness of the environmental and social impact of large schemes in which he was involved convinced him of the need for engineers to resist being pigeon-holed as 'technical experts'. They need to be more proactive in considering the wider implications of their decisions. In his view, the true professional needs the freedom to act in accordance with their own personal judgement, unbiased by the overriding needs of the employer or other external stakeholders. This personal judgement should be informed by wise normative guidelines from a professional body which allows the maintenance of standards and objectivity in complex situations.

Beginning with the historical roots of the Code of Practice of the Institution of Civil Engineers (ICE), he then describes the development of the current code and the way it is used to guide and discipline members. Finally, by way of illustrating the situations to which the Code must be related, he discusses some very interesting examples of the approaches used in large-scale projects where wider social and environmental values have been specifically prioritised.

A couple of more general emergent issues about the relationship between values and professions can be highlighted here.

First, both these chapters raise the issue of the place of formal written value statements and how these are implemented by actual professional practitioners. While the two chapters differ on the extent to which they believe that codes can be directly translated into practice, with Armstrong taking the view that the ICE Code of Practice is a very present help in resolving practical issues and Wainwright and Pattison adopting a more agnostic stance, the point is that the relationship between officially espoused written values and values enacted by practitioners needs to be brought together into some kind of conscious conversation or dialogue. It is not enough for professions to have codes of practice and values. They need to pay attention to possible gaps between ideals and realities in the ways that professionals actually perform, and this in a form other than just using codes as a text against which to discipline deviants.

Implicit in the former point, and emerging from both the chapters, is a clear acknowledgement that written codes with the values they contain need active interpretation in everyday practical situations if they are to be of significance and use. Codes can provide basic values and horizons for action, but without ongoing, active interpretation and deliberation on the part of practitioners they fall into desuetude. For codes to contribute to the preservation and promotion of important professional values, it is not enough that they should simply have been created and exist. They must be constantly correlated with experience, discussed and debated. There is no such thing as a self-interpreting code which makes it clear to practitioners in all times and places what they should do. Rather, codes need critical contextual discernment from the practitioners they are expected to guide. At best, they can help practitioners work with values in practice, but they cannot fully determine how each practitioner might always act. Thus, their universal normativity for professional members is necessarily constrained by the need for individual professionals to exercise proper professional judgement in relation to their practice. Codes therefore form part of the interrogative critical framework for enacting values in practice, not the end of all doubt and uncertainty.

The chapters in this section provide further evidence that the relationship between values and professional practice is a complex and dynamic one. Even at the high point of articulation of values in professional codes, there is much scope for uncertainty and lack of clarity. These two chapters illustrate again the complexities surrounding the issues of values and the uses to which they are put.

CHAPTER 8

What can we expect of professional codes of conduct, practice and ethics?

Paul Wainwright and Stephen Pattison

Introduction

In contemporary society, professional codes abound. In recent years, indeed, they have proliferated. Witness the guidelines for the implementation of the recently published *Code of Conduct for NHS Managers*:

> NHS managers must follow the 'Nolan Principles on Conduct in Public Life', the 'Corporate Governance Codes of Conduct and Accountability', the 'Standards of Business Conduct', the 'Code of Practice on Openness in the NHS' and standards of good employment practice.
>
> (Department of Health 2002: 8)

Codes of conduct, practice and ethics are important sites for the study of values in professional practice, acting as repositories and conveyors of such values. They might well be regarded as the epitome of understanding, defining and articulating occupational purpose, practice and identity. If we want to learn what the values of a profession and its members are, we might reasonably turn to its published code as an authoritative statement. Externally, they indicate to the public and other non members of the profession what they may expect from those who adhere to the code. From the internal perspective they instruct the members of the profession in their duties. Thus the Nursing and Midwifery Council (NMC) in the UK states:

The purpose of the *Code of Professional Conduct* is to:
- inform the professions of the standard of professional conduct required of them in the exercise of their professional account-ability and practice
- inform the public, other professions and employers of the standard of professional conduct that they can expect of a registered practitioner.

(NMC 2002a)

The importance of codes should not be underestimated. Codes are used to hold individual members of professions to account. They may have statutory or quasi-statutory functions in terms of the removal of the right to practise. They provide a standard when assessing allegations of misconduct or malpractice. They also have to do with the negotiation of the mandate and licence of a profession, serving as a profession's declaration of its values and aspirations and restricting its actions. Codes often function as a teaching resource, transmitting fundamental ideas about values from one generation of practitioners to the next, and helping shape identity and practice. Codes might, and arguably should, stimulate ethical reflection, although whether they aid moral decision making is more debatable (Pattison 2001).

At a certain stage in the development of any substantial occupational group, there often arises an impetus to codify in writing the basic principles, values, attitudes and orientations that can be expected of members of that group by their colleagues and clients. The codes that emerge might be expected to be authoritative, coherent statements and guidelines that will reflect, shape and express professional identity and behaviour in a clear, unambiguous way.

A superficial inspection of such documents often suggests that they should perform just this function. They are usually produced with the full authority of the professional body, guaranteed by corporate logos. They have the full weight of anonymous corporate authorship, without any hint that their production might have involved dispute and discussion. The principles and guidelines that they commend are often presented as timelessly valid, uncontroversial and consistent. *Prima facie,* these codes look and function a bit like scripture in some religions. Like the Bible, also regarded as an authoritative, timeless document by many Christians, codes, while they may not be read daily by professional members, may be held to be a helpful back-ground document which, when problems arise, will resolve difficulties about practising as a professional or receiving professional services.

If codes in their form, content and usage are taken to have some of the qualities of identity-forming, totemic, quasi-religious scriptures, perhaps they deserve some of the criticism to which scriptures have been exposed. Here, we want to suggest that codes are less straightforward and more contradic-tory and interesting documents than they appear at first sight. There are many theoretical and practical problems associated with their content and usage.

Referring mainly to the codes used in the health sector, we want to explore some of the difficulties, contradictions and shortcomings of these lapidary-seeming documents. Our overall argument is that people expect both too much and too little from codes, often assuming meaning, clarity and unity that is not there. Unfortunately, the codes often lend themselves to this kind of confusion, for reasons which will become clear as we proceed.

If the first impression gained from codes is that they are simple, monolithic documents, like a kind of secular 'Ten Commandments', metaphorically inscribed on tablets of stone, we hope to show here that they are dynamic and confusing artefacts that directly, but tacitly, reflect the clashes of values and interests of those engaged in complex work in a complex ecology of values and principles within and outside the particular occupational groups to which they pertain. Far from being tablets of stone, they are more like the shiny balls that hang, rotating, from the ceilings of discotheques, reflecting and refracting professional values from different perspectives. Like scriptures, they require active interpretation by the individuals and groups who read and put them into operation (Edgar 2003).

Codes are characterised by a mixture of the reflective and the imperative, the aspirational and the descriptive, the ethical and the pragmatic. They are not clear, unambiguous unified expressions of enacted consensual values. We want to suggest that because of their internal contradictions and tensions, they are not able to perform the function that people perhaps most expect of them, i.e. precisely to determine professional values and practice in a direct, immediate, quotidian way. Instead, they represent unfinished, confused interim statements that reflect the horizons of professional and social conflicts about values in the context of complex working situations. While they may be able to set loose boundaries of discourse on the nature of values in professional practice, they cannot resolve the ambiguities of active values management facing practitioners engaged in multivalent situations where professional judgement is required to make an adequate response.

Cantwell Smith suggests that 'People – a given community – make a text into scripture, or keep it scripture, by treating it in a certain way' (Cantwell Smith 1993: 181). He goes on to argue that 'scripture is human activity', i.e. an active ongoing process, not a single event or document. It is precisely this dynamic understanding of codes as unfinished, ongoing activity which, in this discussion, we want to insert into the expectations of these documents. This should serve to make usage and discussion more complex and more realistic in the context of understanding the expression and operationalisation of professional values in codes.

We now go on selectively to examine some of the factors that often make professional codes ambiguous and difficult vehicles for professional values.

Authorship and creation

Confusion and ambiguity about the nature and content of codes begins with their authorship and construction. Published codes are usually anonymous and do not explain their own origins and construction. This means that they present as consensual documents without sectional interest or prejudice. They may indeed be so. However, as with the understanding or interpretation of any text, it is worth asking questions of authorship and construction and their implications. Ultimately, all codes reflect someone's interests and values as well as their ideas about desirable practice and professional control.

In the case of at least some codes, authorship may well be wholly or mainly the work of one enthusiast who regards the code as important. Reg Pyne, a senior nurse, was one such whose commitment was decisive in shaping the first version of the United Kingdom Central Council for Nursing, Midwifery and Health Visiting (UKCC) Code of Professional Conduct. (The UKCC was the predecessor of the current NMC.)

Sometimes, enthusiasts are supported by a working group or committee. However, it is unusual for a whole profession to be extensively involved in the shaping of a code. It is even more unusual for members of the public to have a voice in shaping it. The consequence is that many codes, while appearing to command universal support for consensual principles and values, may actually be rather partial documents reflecting particular interests, e.g. those of the 'top' professionals who wish to have a measure of control over their juniors.

This is not to denigrate particular codes. It is just to point out that codes do not spring fully formed out of nowhere, and that some interests and values may be emphasised while other values on the edges of the profession may be marginalised or ignored. None of which would matter but for the fact that codes usually present themselves – and are claimed by those who have recourse to them – as speaking in a general voice for a whole profession.

Explicit and implicit dimensions

Like many written documents, codes are often not as unambiguous and clear as they may at first appear to be. Many texts harbour implicit subtexts or ideologies that tacitly commend a particular view of the world or a specific set of values. Sometimes these subtexts may be more important than many of the explicit and overt principles set out in the code. So, for example, many codes have high ethical principles in them such as the need to promote autonomy and to respect clients. However, these important moral principles may be put on a par with other values such as preserving the good name and reputation of the profession and not bringing it into disrepute. It is possible to interpret some codes as being more concerned with the well-being of the profession than its clients (e.g. Hunt 1994). This is not something that is likely to be highlighted and made very overt. It does, however, represent a real potential for a clash of values in the form and usage of codes that sometimes becomes a practical problem for practitioners and users of professional services. The import of all this is that readers and users of codes need to be self-consciously aware of the covert and marginal significance and meanings of these texts and should not just be impressed by the high moral principles and rhetoric that are likely to form at least part of these documents.

Different functions for codes

According to Hussey (1996: 252), codes of conduct have seven functions:

- guidance – in the course of professional work
- regulation – prescribing norms of behaviour, moral standards and values
- discipline – allowing transgressions to be identified and sanctions imposed
- protection – protecting the public who rely on the professional services, and protecting the employers who employ professionals
- information – telling clients, colleagues, etc. what standards to expect, and therefore promoting trust
- proclamation – telling the world that a group of workers aspires to professional status
- negotiation – serving to justify a stance or course of action, which may be in dispute.

Unfortunately, these functions are not usually explicitly set out or discussed in published codes, nor are the tensions and contradictions between different functions explored. They mostly remain implicit. Furthermore, the writers of particular codes may not have considered the range of functions that they wish these documents to fulfil. Therefore, there is always the possibility that they themselves may be surprised by the uses to which their work can be put.

If people do not consciously consider and circumscribe the nature of the codes they construct, it is not difficult to see that there can be considerable scope for clashes and tensions between the various functions outlined above. So, for example, if a code that is primarily intended to provide general guiding principles is used to discipline people on specific issues, it may be that its guidance function is vitiated because professional members will want it to be tightened up and made more legal in its tone and concerns. If one is to be judged and perhaps face disqualification from practice, it is natural to expect explicit criteria against which the judgement is to be made.

Choosing the functions of a code, then administering and policing them, is an activity that reflects a set of values and principles in itself. If this is not done very consciously, then certain treasured professional values might be undermined from the start. So, for example, an overprescriptive, legalistic code may militate against the creation of autonomous individual professionals who are encouraged to use and take responsibility for their own individual judgements about complex work.

Impossible ideals?

Codes often contain a requirement to respect some very important fundamental values and principles, such as to 'act always in such a manner as to promote and safeguard the interests and well-being of patients and clients' (UKCC 1992: Clause 1). Unfortunately, it is often not practically possible to maintain such values within everyday professional life and, as Hussey (1996) suggests, they are frequently so broadly drawn as to be attractive but of no practical help. So these values and principles can represent problematic ideals.

A recent comparison of nursing codes of conduct in six European countries (European Council of Nursing 2002) suggested that the ethical principle of autonomy is discussed in most such codes. As the principle of autonomy rests on the notion of respect for persons, this must refer to the autonomy of both the nurse as an independent professional practitioner and to the patient as a recipient of care and treatment. However, no professional practitioner working in a healthcare institution is exempt from the restrictions on their autonomy imposed by an employer through the contract of employment. Furthermore, professionals are bound by legal statutes and the limitations of their licence to practise.

At the informal level, in the healthcare team there is an imbalance of power and authority between members of the same, and of different, professions. For MacIntyre (1981), it is a requirement of participation in a practice that practitioners submit to the superior expertise and authority of those more skilled than they. This inevitably requires the occasional loss of autonomy. Most health professionals find themselves implicitly or explicitly dominated by the power and authority of the medical profession. This means that their autonomy is substantially and routinely restricted. Patients, too, have their autonomy unavoidably curtailed, not least by the mere fact of admission to a hospital.

Confidentiality is another explicit and implicit requirement of most codes for professionals who work in some interpersonal contexts with clients. Observing this cardinal principle is, however, beset with problems. Clients must share relevant information with professionals if they are to receive an effective service. This may require the reassurance of a confidential relationship. However, professionals will often need to pass this information on to others, either because of their involvement in the team responsible for the service, or for more complicated reasons. Most health service users expect that information given to a doctor or a nurse will become shared with other health professionals. Codes of conduct are a powerful way of formalising the network of restricted, confidential disclosure. However, it is not always so easy to keep information within the team.

Take, for example, the 13-year-old girl with severe abdominal pain, admitted to the emergency department. An important investigation, in the absence of more obvious pathology, would be a pregnancy test to exclude the possibility of an ectopic pregnancy. It is a regrettably common occurrence for a 13-year-old to become pregnant, and an ectopic pregnancy is a life-threatening condition. However, the need to carry out the test and to inform the patient and others, such as her parents, of the result can lead to a variety of consequences, as would any decision to keep the facts confidential to the medical team. Even the limitations of the built environment in wards, emergency departments and consulting rooms result in inevitable, accidental degradation of privacy and confidentiality for patients and their families.

There are many other examples of individual requirements of codes causing difficulties: requirements for consent, truth telling, privacy, virtue, duty and collaboration all feature in the codes reviewed for the European study and each will have internal conflicts and contradictions.

Contradictions between values and principles

Equally problematic is the potential for conflict between two or more main guiding principles or fundamental values in codes. For example, recently nurses have been concerned that the UK ruling body for nursing agreed that the covert administration of medicines by nurses to elderly patients was acceptable in certain circumstances. On the one hand, nurses are usually committed to obtaining proper consent to treatment, and to being open and honest in their dealings with patients. However, they also have obligations to administer prescribed medication, and to treat the patient in ways that could be said to be in the patient's interests.

If there are good grounds for supposing that the patient needs the medication and if there is some doubt about the patient's competence, perhaps if they are confused or suffering from dementia, there will be a strong desire to administer the therapy. If a confused patient, suffering from Alzheimer's disease, physically resists taking medication, it is tempting to assume that they are not making a competent refusal. This would allow the nurse to treat without consent, acting in the patient's best interests. However, a physical struggle with the patient, to forcibly administer the drug either orally or by injection, is distressing for all concerned: the patient, the nurses, other patients, and any relatives or others who may observe the situation. How much better, then, to crush the pill or break open the capsule, mix it with some pleasant drink, or in some bread and jam, and dupe the patient into accepting it.

But what if the medication in question is a sedative or tranquilliser, and what if the primary motivation is to quieten a noisy and restless patient at bedtime? It could be argued that the patient is distressed and will be happier if sedated. Furthermore, noisy, confused patients are distressing for other patients and create considerable workload for over-stretched nurses. However, a patient with dementia may be distressed because in moments of lucidity they are frightened and distressed by what is happening. And such a patient may well dislike intensely the sensation of being drugged, and far from relaxing into a comfortably sedated sleep, they may suffer hallucinations or have nightmares.

If the code of conduct enjoins nurses to respect the autonomy and dignity of patients, to act always so as to put their interests first, to maintain a safe and proper therapeutic environment for all those in their care, and to comply with medical instructions, it is difficult to see how even the best nurse can be in compliance with all the demands of the code.

Similar dilemmas will frequently arise in other healthcare situations, such as when making decisions about whether or not to resuscitate older patients or very premature infants, whether to initiate or continue with artificial feeding regimes for brain-injured patients, how to manage increasingly distressing symptoms in the terminal stages of motor neurone disease, and many others.

Nurses are not the only professionals in the health sector who must cope with such tensions. The *Code of Conduct for NHS Managers* states that the manager will:

> ... support and assist the Accountable Officer of my organisation in his or her responsibility to answer to Parliament, Ministers and the Department of Health in terms of fully and faithfully declaring and explaining the use of resources and the performance of the local NHS in putting national policy into practice and delivering targets.
>
> (Department of Health 2002: 6)

However, it also states that managers will:

- make the care and safety of patients their first concern and act to protect them from risk
- respect the public, patients, relatives, carers, NHS staff and partners in other agencies (Department of Health 2002: 4).

This contradictory guidance makes it very unclear where a manager's primary responsibilities and loyalties should really lie. There would seem to be clear scope for conflicts between these injunctions. (For more on the responsibilities and duties of healthcare managers, *see* Chapter 5.)

In whose interests?

Professions like to present codes as embodying the value of seeking the benefit of the public. However, members of the public generally have little say in the contents or administration of codes. Indeed, they frequently do not know that they exist. If they do access them, they may well find it hard to become clear as to their rights in relation to them (Pattison 2001). In a number of cases, action which might have been to the public benefit either for individuals or groups has actually been inhibited by the implementation of codes. We have already mentioned that preserving the good reputation of the profession can take precedence over ethical principles like preserving individual autonomy of patients or seeking justice for a group.

To stay with the example of nursing, the UKCC, and its predecessor the General Nursing Council, always maintained emphatically that their primary role was the protection of the public, not the representation or protection of the profession. However, the application of the UKCC Code has not always seemed to serve the value of preserving public interest well.

Witness the widely publicised case concerning a charge nurse called Graham Pink. In 1989, Pink complained about the level of staffing and quality of care in an older people's ward on which he worked. He began by writing to his health authority employers. When he received no satisfaction, he wrote various letters and articles in the press. He was eventually dismissed by his employers and began an action for unfair dismissal. This was eventually settled out of court in 1992 (http://www.freedomtocare.org/page73.htm). Not only did he feel that he had failed to achieve the improvements he sought, he suffered considerable hardship. He tried, in his view, to use the UKCC Code of Conduct to support his actions but was disappointed that, although the UKCC rejected an accusation of misconduct against him, it did little or nothing to support him. He is quoted as saying, 'I have upheld the [UKCC] Code [of Conduct] religiously, and as a result I face losing my job ... I see it as a very negative force at the moment ... it certainly doesn't do any good for patients' (Cole 1991).

However, to criticise codes for failing to bring to book unsatisfactory care organisations, such as health trusts or hospitals, while highlighting a real limitation and possible flaw in terms of promoting professional values, is perhaps to miss the point. In its disciplinary function, the code is intended to protect the public against the vicious or incompetent individual practitioner.

A professional regulatory body such as the UKCC, NMC or General Medical Council (GMC) has no relationship with, and no authority over, organisations. They stand between the individual practitioner and the individual member of the public and there must be a specific accusation of misconduct against a practitioner before they can act. However, if failures in an organisation result from the professional misconduct of a member of the profession *who happens also to be a manager*, then that individual professional can be disciplined and struck off for their personal conduct, as happened in the case of the Chief Executive of Bristol Children's' Hospital following revelations about paediatric cardiac surgery services (HMSO 2001).

NHS managers and clinicians

An interesting distinction may be made here between the codes set out by bodies responsible for professional conduct and licensure, such as the NMC, the GMC or the Law Society, and the *Code of Conduct for NHS Managers*. The latter was introduced as part of the Department of Health response to the Kennedy Report (HMSO 2001) of the inquiry into the Bristol heart surgery scandal. It was produced, published and implemented by the Department of Health (albeit after a prolonged period of negotiation and development by the Institute of Healthcare Management), and was introduced by a letter from the Chief Executive of the NHS. It is thus a management tool, used to discipline employees of the organisation that produced it. It is to be incorporated into the contract of employment of senior NHS managers, but carries no sanctions equivalent to the removal of a professional's right to practise. (*See also* Chapter 5.)

Codes as detailed guidance for practitioners

We have suggested that codes may often be perceived as normative, prescriptive tools for the regulation of professional practice. However, we have also suggested that codes may not be quite the everyday working documents that one might suppose. Is a code something that is set in some sort of robust framework, and which is then used as a regular source for everyday reference? Is a professional code something that every practitioner should have on laminated plastic in their wallets? Should they publicly sign up to a code, as some people have to with the code of conduct for local government or the code of conduct for ministers, or have it written into their contracts, like the NHS managers' code? When practitioners admit to not knowing much about their profession's code, should we be surprised and worried? These questions go to the heart of the debate about the use and function of codes.

Anecdotally, when one asks nurses about the UKCC Code, they say they only refer to it in dispute situations. It is used in situations of crisis and employment dispute rather than as an everyday companion to virtuous behaviour. The NMC mailed the new edition of their code to every one of the 600 000 or so nurses on the professional register. However, when nurses were asked, casually, whether they knew about it, many said that they did not (European Council of Nursing 2002). In the light of this kind of usage and experience, it would be interesting to know whether this relative ignorance and neglect is consonant with the hopes and intentions of code-formulating professional bodies and authors.

Hussey (1996: 252) summarises some of the practical problems in using codes. In particular, he notes that they 'fail to give practical guidance either in matters of general morality or on the special issues thrown up by professional duties'. Tadd has specifically argued that the (then) UKCC Code did not enhance the moral climate of nursing or raise standards of care, and that it did not empower nurses (Tadd 1994). However, as Hussey points out, there are considerable difficulties in attempting to produce a code that could achieve any of these objectives, other than in a very general way (Hussey 1996).

Codes, like other writings, are not self-implementing. They can achieve nothing by and of themselves. Practitioners, together with their professional leaders and educators, bear the main responsibility for ensuring an appropriate moral climate and standards of care within everyday practice. Continual reference to the rule book can make effective, responsive professional performance impossible. It conflicts with the spirit of many of the codes themselves. These aim to outline general principles but to locate responsibility for judgement in specific complex cases firmly with the competent professional.

Codes frequently exhort practitioners to be honest, or trustworthy, or to act with integrity. This represents an appeal to moral virtue (*see*, for example, Foot 1978; Gardiner 2003). Leaving aside the problem of whether a code can *require* practitioners to be virtuous (Pattison 2001), the point about the moral virtues is that virtuous people will decide for themselves what to do in specific situations, allowing their sense of honesty, or integrity, or justice to direct their actions. No set of rules or clauses in a code can tell us how to act with compassion or courage, still less what amounts to the best interests of any given patient.

The incessant demand, from some practitioners and some critics of codes, for codes to be effective in guiding daily practice sounds a bit like the immature complaints of children in the schoolyard demanding that the rules be set out and followed down to the minutest detail in a game of tag. In failing to provide specific answers to specific problems, codes are no different from theories of ethics. Codes and ethical theories can both offer some general principles to apply to our problems, but they cannot solve them for us.

What can we expect of professional codes?

There are all kinds of theoretical and practical problems with codes. Professional codes are much more complex and ambivalent documents with regard to professional values and practice than they may have seemed at first. In particular, they do not tell us much specifically about practice, and perhaps they should not be expected to do so.

If we want to know why doctors and nurses do what they do, why it is that women managed in maternity care by midwives are less likely to have caesareans or epidurals than women managed by doctors, why it is that patients seen by the nurse practitioner are more likely to know what is wrong with them than those seen by the doctor, why it is that doctors may pay little attention to the story told them by the patient and more attention to the pathology results (e.g. Jewson 1976; Watts *et al.* 2002), we may have to examine their values. However, they are unlikely to be the kind of values we will find in a code of conduct.

Codes cannot capture all, or even most, that is worth knowing about professional practice. Indeed, they may be antithetical to recognising what is really important in professional activity. Schon's (1984) critique of the failure of the technical–rational approach to solve the complex problems that confront professionals suggests that attempts to codify our responses are of little use in the unique and complex encounter between professional and client. Noddings has also argued that the caring response must, necessarily, be unpredictable (Noddings 1984).

We suggested at the outset that codes might be seen by many as coherent, monolithic and authoritative repositories or expressions of the values of a profession. We have gone on to argue that they are problematic at best, and that they cannot and should not fulfil the purpose for which some commentators and stakeholders think they should be used.

Codes are not univocal, uncontroversial guides to all aspects of attitude, orientation, identity and behaviour that resolve questions of value for professionals. Rather, they can be seen as emergent, living documents-in-creation that reflect the mixed and conflicted value ecology of society in general as well as particular occupational cultures within the social order. Codes are not incontrovertible, non-controversial documents that bring a closure to confusion and debate. In many ways they reflect and in some ways add to it within the context of complex professional work.

All this means that authors, publishers and users of codes, whether members of professions or consumers of their services, need to have a much more realistic view of the nature and functions of these documents. We need to have realistic attitudes and expectations of professional codes.

Some conclusions

The discussion above suggests the following.

First, codes cannot be expected to address or resolve all practical and theoretical problems. They may represent a useful contribution to thinking about practice and informing the reflection of practitioners engaged in complex work that requires specific personal judgements. But they cannot provide a substitute for that judgement. Thus, they cannot provide comforting dogma or closure for professionals working through value conflicts in everyday life. Indeed, if properly considered, they may even exacerbate those conflicts.

Secondly, given that written codes basically represent unfinished, ongoing reflections of value conflicts and negotiations emerging from living social relationships amongst groups and individuals, it is important that all those groups and individuals affected by them should take some responsibility for these documents. If codes are to be dethroned and demystified so they are seen as contingent and living human creations, this means that those who live within their ambit should not try to hide behind an anonymous text, but rather should seek to become active authors and interpreters of the values that are found therein. Scriptures are dead and distorted if they are regarded as being complete without living human beings who embody, interpret and, if necessary, rewrite them. Generally, more people need to take more active responsibility for the writing, implementation and interpretation of the values implicit in codes as part of being active professionals. Professional values as expressed in codes should be the real, espoused and enacted values of many, not just the aspirations of an élite few.

Finally, underlying both the previous points is the general view that professionals might need to become much more self-consciously responsible 'value managers', both within their everyday practice and corporately as members of particular occupational groups whose conflicted values are set out in codes. If codes do not resolve value conflicts in everyday practice and reflect different possible values requiring judgements and choices, then there is a great need for professionals, individually and corporately, to give them a good deal more active critical attention.

If such critical attention and responsibility is taken by professionals, this can only help codes to become much better reflections of values within specific occupational ranks and also the basis for active positive value discussion. If codes come to be perceived much more directly as interim, imperfect, active documents for dispute, discussion and ongoing reformulation, they will no longer be half-forgotten reference pieces that are only dusted off in times of crisis. They will become a real resource for professional reflection and self-conscious identity formation in partnership with others. This can only be to the good given the amount of time and effort that goes into shaping documents that presently are often perceived as the dead letter of the law, filed under the category 'take no action'. Unfortunately, the very way by which codes currently get developed, formalised and promulgated, through statutory, regulatory bodies, could hardly be more precisely calculated to prevent the kind of dynamic approach that we would advocate.

Codes represent very imperfect, contradictory and unsatisfactory tools for value reinforcement and reproduction. For all that, they have real value. They form a necessary if not sufficient starting point for reflecting on values in professional practice. But if they are to have a larger, more positive role in nurturing and expressing virtues, rather than just being used somewhat *ad hoc* to police particular practices, they probably need to be more porous and creative documents that must be reconstrued in terms of clarity, purpose and, particularly, use. Codes need to become living scripture, in Cantwell Smith's (1993) sense of the term, rather than dead dogma.

CHAPTER 9

The development and use of codes of practice for professional engineers

James Armstrong

Introduction

As a practising civil engineer, graduating from Glasgow University in 1946, I have had the satisfaction of taking part in many major projects, mostly as a design consultant. I retired in 1990 as a senior partner of a large multi-disciplinary consultancy consisting of planners, architects, engineers and surveyors. My experience included major development projects and studies; these ranged from shopping centres, teaching hospitals and university buildings to the terminal works for the Channel Tunnel and the new airport in the Falkland Islands. I was the senior partner responsible for overseas work for several years, visiting many countries in the Middle and Far East. I have taken an active interest in our professional organisations throughout my career, becoming President of the Institution of Structural Engineers in 1990. I am a Fellow of the senior learned society, the Royal Academy of Engineering and have sat on many committees and working parties over many years.

My interest in professional ethics and values was stimulated by my overseas work, and by having to consider fundamental issues, rather than accepting my own national and cultural norms as universal (Armstrong *et al.* 1999).

A personal perspective on values and ethics for engineers

Ethical decisions are concerned specifically with quality – with justice, with equity, with the consequences for all affected by the decision, with the personal and collective responsibilities which lie beyond the contractual obligations into which we enter. In complex developed societies, certain functions requiring special knowledge and responsibilities, which affect the quality of life for others, are described as professional, and the duties are defined and monitored.

Making a decision requires an evaluation of alternative courses of action with reference to a set of basic values. In this chapter I will explore the decision-making responsibilities of professional engineers, and the structures that they have put in place to help them respond appropriately.

Decision making in practice

Engineers frequently make big decisions. They can create greater well-being or long-term problems for society. Roman road builders had a longer-lasting influence upon the shape of society than their emperors' wars. Irrigation projects built 1800 years ago in northern Sri Lanka are still serving the inhabitants faithfully.

Technical and political changes are taking place more rapidly now than at any time in the past. The scale and range of societies, the size of projects undertaken by them – projects concerned with education, healthcare, government, public and private works, and many other areas of communal concern – have greatly increased over those undertaken in previous centuries.

These developments result in the need to recognise that world communities are becoming much more interdependent. Differing views as to acceptable values held in common by a society have a very real impact upon our quality of life. The decisions of a single individual can affect the lives of many millions of others – for better or worse.

The contemporary ethical situation is one of confusion. There is no single vision or definition of the 'common good'. There is a stress on liberalism (the individual can think or do what he likes provided it doesn't interfere with the freedom of another) and pluralism (the acceptance of many different views about what is good.)

Ethical decisions involve concepts of duty and responsibility of conflicts between rival goods or ills. We each develop a personal value system influenced by the social and cultural norms of our environment. The framework of value and ethical decision making can be conceived as having three main aspects:

- our personal conditioning and values
- the structure and values of the community in which we live
- the scale and range of the effects of the decisions we make.

Our personal 'conditioning' is based on our individual upbringing and culture. It is also influenced by our individual talents, perhaps for music, mathematics, language, leadership or service. It is useful to explore our personal beliefs from time to time, to consider whether these are fundamental or merely relative.

Our decisions are also influenced by the customs and laws of the societies in which we live. Some of these are enshrined in the culture, others are defined in the body of common law or as statutes. Careful consideration of these social norms is needed before making any major decision, particularly if it is likely to affect a significant number of people. Beyond the limits of the nation state and its laws and sanctions lie humanity and justice – this sphere of influence is now more relevant because of the growing international dimension of today's relationships. If we consider our own position as responsible members of the human race, then on whose behalf are we acting? Our duty is to care for the creation – not only for our immediate family or circle of friends and colleagues.

The third aspect of ethical behaviour is concerned with the consequences of our actions, their range and duration. These can be limited to ourselves or our immediate family, but they can also have wider effects. They can affect humanity or even creation as a whole. Major construction projects, for example, sometimes affect the quality of life of many people for decades, if not centuries – indeed, it is often intended that they should. They can cause major disasters. A hierarchy of consequences can therefore be set out:

- What is good for me?
- What is good for society?
- What is good for humanity?
- What is good for creation?

Engineers are concerned with balanced judgements, requiring understanding and independent evaluations. They need to know which decisions are likely to produce the most favourable results, both in the short and in the longer term. Reflections upon the ethical significance and correctness of any situation require the use of judgemental reason, which needs to be fine-tuned to the overall needs of society and not merely to the use of deductive logic and the pursuit of the 'correct' answer to technical problems.

Problems that arise in everyday practice

Problems in practice with ethical and value dimensions rarely have a single solution. They evolve in complex relationships and are part of a continuum whose components are inextricably entwined with one another. In dealing with such problems, it is not possible to provide precise rules and regulations, only to suggest guidelines. It is this that gives ethical behaviour its special place in maintaining the quality of life in the professions. It distinguishes ethical behaviour from lawful behaviour, which follows clearly defined positive instructions evolved by a society to curb antisocial behaviour. There is thus often a clear distinction between social regulation and personal professional responsibility.

The challenge which professional engineers face is to relate reflective moral thought and personal values and choices to the context of national and international laws and conventions.

The role of the practising professional

One definition of profession provided by the *Concise Oxford Dictionary* (1964) is 'a vocation, a calling, one requiring advanced knowledge or training in some branch of learning or science'.

The professional is a client's agent, not a servant. To be a member of a profession is to:

- have specialised knowledge and skill
- have power – the power of knowledge and the capacity to affect society
- have undergone a period of training, which includes skills but also the development of reason
- be a member of a professional body which is responsible for regulating standards, protecting rights of practice, ensuring proper training and for maintaining the correct professional behaviour of its members.

According to Bennion (1969), professional practitioners of all disciplines are said to need six qualities:

- integrity – openness and honesty, both with themselves and with others
- independence – freedom from secondary interests with other parties
- impartiality – freedom from bias and unbalanced interests
- responsibility – the recognition and acceptance of personal commitment
- competence – a thorough knowledge of the work they undertake
- discretion – care with communications, trustworthiness.

These personal qualities enable the maintenance of principles and responsibilities in professional activities in contexts which are often complex and unclear. Not least, with growing specialisation in the division of work, there is the danger of the 'expert' becoming focused purely on technical matters. This can affect the professional's perception, discouraging holistic thinking and inhibiting the full understanding of the context of professional work. I will now elaborate more specifically on the importance of these qualities in professional work.

Integrity implies the discovery and communication of the truth in such a way as to enable the client and others to make informed decisions. Honesty and integrity are essential for the development of trust.

Independence denotes freedom from any special interest group. To be involved with either an employer or an action group in such a way that judgement is clouded is to lose professional autonomy. By virtue of specialist knowledge the professional has an intrinsic authority. Extrinsic authority is also vested in professionals by virtue of the positions that they hold.

Impartiality enables professionals to fulfil their duties to clients and to treat all parties equally. There is a need to avoid self-interest, or the interest of one's employing firm, which may equally cloud professional judgement.

Responsibility involves the realistic assessment of skills and the acceptance of limitations. The professional acknowledges the responsibilities of others, accepts personal responsibility and works as part of a team. The engineer has a duty of care for the general public, for the users of the project, for the peer group of professional engineers and for clients and employers.

Most members of the construction industry are now 'professionals'. Consultants are concerned externally with meeting the needs of their clients, and internally with the commercial aspects of their practice, with marketing and fee-bidding strategies. Contractors are leading teams of 'professionals' in management contracts and in design-and-build contracts.

Roles are sometimes combined with those of financial and legal specialists in modern private finance initiative (PFI) projects, to finance, design, build, operate and hand over projects. This interweaving of roles requires an awareness of the responsibilities of professionals. It is difficult to maintain responsibilities as an 'agent', rather than as a 'contractor', during the very close relationships arising during a total procurement process. Professionals are still responsible for making decisions that others have not the skills and training to make. The need for integrity, independence, impartiality and responsibility is even greater. The responsibility for one's role in collaborative work within and beyond the profession is of prime importance.

Competence requires a duty to seek appropriate training and experience. It is essential to the fulfilment of professional responsibilities to society. The ethical requirement is in the acknowledgement of the need to be competent, rather than in the competence itself. Skills can be misused. An essential element of professional practice is the capacity to reflect upon, to evaluate and to accept different levels of competence, and to ensure that the necessary skill is deployed, even if it has to be provided by others.

Discretion is essential in the maintenance of trust. Information must be treated on a 'need to know' basis, and not transmitted unnecessarily to others. In some cases, on defence projects for example, consultants will be under an agreement not to divulge information to others. However, if they are seriously concerned about the consequences of some action, professionals must also be able to raise matters of concern with clients and, if necessary, with higher authorities.

The importance of professional bodies

The existence of an institution or formal body of professionals is essential to the preservation and promotion of appropriate professional qualities, proper conduct and competent decision making. Such a body is responsible for the development and maintenance of professional values and competencies. It will enable and encourage professionals to reflect upon their own integrity and to learn from the experience of others, as well as transmitting professional culture over generations. It provides an external but informed perspective, which enables proper reflection and responsibility.

It should be noted that the quality of integrity, important for individual professionals, is not confined to those individuals. It is a vital corporate requirement for professional institutions and management groups. The profession as a whole has to be consistent and to be able to relate values to practice. Without this, the recognition of the profession as a body of experts concerned for public welfare will be eroded. With that will go the trust essential to the functioning of any professional relationship. The professional body must also avoid the moral ambiguity of acting as a body protecting the interests of its individual members. It is not a trade union or trade association, it is a body concerned to ensure the highest standards of professional service to the community.

In the case of professional engineering, the Institution of Civil Engineers (ICE) is the main professional body. This originated in 1771 as a dining club of civil engineers. It was formally constituted as an Institution in 1817 with the inaugural meeting being held on 2 January 1818. In his address on that occasion, Henry Palmer described the Institution as:

> A Society for the general advancement of Mechanical Science and more particularly for promoting the acquisition of that species of knowledge which constitutes the profession of a Civil Engineer, being the art of directing the Great Sources of Power in Nature for the use and convenience of man ....
> (Original Charter of Incorporation of the ICE, 1828)

The ICE now:

- acts as a learned society, advancing the science and technology of engineering
- sets standards for professional education and training
- regulates the practice of the individual professional
- enables the professional development of moral awareness, skills and responsibility
- provides support for professionals in decision making and areas of conflicts of interest
- plays a major role in communicating with the public.

The practice of engineering

> The Engineer is a Mediator between the Philosopher and the Working Mechanic, and like an interpreter between two

foreigners, must understand the language of both, hence the absolute necessity of possessing both practical and theoretical knowledge.

(Henry Palmer, inaugural address of the ICE, 2 January 1818 [Watson 1988: 9])

If Palmer's definition of the engineer is accepted then the professional engineer, acting as such, can never truly be an employee. The true professional needs and retains the freedom to act in accordance with personal judgement, unbiased by the overriding needs of any employer. As a project manager, an engineer may be held to have an overriding loyalty to the company, to its efficiency and profitability. As a professional, however, the engineer has responsibilities for the wider interests of safety, health and welfare of the public and the protection of the environment. This can produce conflicts of interest, requiring a broad view of their role.

Civil engineering projects are multifaceted. They are complex, unique and built to strict deadlines of cost, time and quality. They are of high value and the result of team effort, often involving inexperienced clients. These constraints require detailed co-ordination and project management, which is often undertaken by the professional engineer.

The engineer's technical skills must be augmented by skills involving human relationships, administration, information management, programming, financial reporting and control, and quality management. The professional engineer serves society. This gives a particular social status, demanding autonomy of decision making to ensure that matters of expediency or finance do not compromise judgement. The engineer can thus be seen as a custodian of the concerns of many different groups of individuals or interests, including the environment and those who have no present voice, even future generations.

Of course, the engineer has to survive and the engineering company needs profits in order to exist. However, the engineer cannot operate simply in a market-orientated way. The creative work of the engineer is not simply a product. It involves a great deal of skill not available to the lay person. The professional engineer is not simply selling services in the market, with the buyer being responsible for deciding between different products (*caveat emptor* – let the buyer beware). Rather engineers offer services, with the buyer needing to trust engineers' skills and judgement (*credat emptor* – let the buyer trust).

The evolution of the ICE Code of Practice

Professional codes are a means of developing the integrity of the professional body. The public declaration of the principles and views on responsibility and practice of a professional organisation provides a benchmark against which the practice of the profession can be evaluated. The role of the professional institution requires that it sets out the relationships between ethical practice and national and international laws and regulations, within the context of cultural diversity and potential conflicts of interest.

In the early years of the ICE and, indeed, in the preceding decades in the eighteenth century, the engineers concerned with major construction works – canals and railways – were well aware of their responsibilities towards society. In a letter written by Smeaton, one of the founder members of the profession, in 1768, he said: 'I have never trusted my reputation in business out of my own hand, so my profession is as perfectly personal as that of any Physician or Counsellor-at-law' (Watson 1988: 6).

This tradition continued and became accepted as a significant aspect of the professional ethos. The first formal iteration of a code of practice for members seems to have been developed in about 1960. A special disciplinary board was established in 1963. Prior to that, complaints about the malpractice of members had been heard before a full meeting of council.

At the instigation of the President of the day, the late Edward Hambly, the ICE conducted a review of its Rules of Practice in 1996/7 with a panel of experienced engineers and lay members. The redrafted code was accepted in 1998. All members of the ICE are required to accept an obligation to follow the Rules of Practice on election to the Institution. If they are found guilty of breaching these Rules then they may be required to resign. The Revised Rules of the ICE (2001) are set out at the end of this chapter.

Prior to 2001, the Rules of the ICE focused upon the interests of clients and fellow professionals. However, the changing context of practice required a review of this traditional emphasis. There was a need to enhance professional standards and to increase awareness of the changing perceptions of the community at large as to the nature of professional integrity and practices. Environmental and human issues, the interests of minority groups, international competition and the growth of information technology all affect our activities. There is an increasing awareness of the importance of regulations about these issues.

The new Rules of Conduct of the Institution were grouped into three categories:

- *General issues.* Responsibilities for the effects of engineering work on the global environment include not only major issues of 'global warming', energy conservation, land use, etc., but also economic issues, such as employment, source of materials, etc.
- *Societal issues.* Responsibilities for the quality of life of other human beings – this would cover disturbance to local populations and all business transactions. Four issues were identified as important: communication, fidelity, practice standards and commercial transactions.
- *Professional issues.* These are responsibilities to fellow professionals, which include upholding the profession's status and ensuring competence and the appropriate transfer of skills from generation to generation.

Some key features concerning integrity and the public interest, from the point of view of the drafting of codes of conduct, are as follows:

- The adoption of a balanced, disciplined and comprehensive approach to problem solving. It should be clear to all that professional judgement and skill are being used to enhance human welfare and to diminish negative effects of developments.
- It must be clear that public functions will be discharged reasonably and lawfully. Conflicts of interest must be avoided; advice must be independent and impartial, free from any personal interests.
- As far as possible, information should be freely available. It should not be used to mislead or deceive, nor should confidential material be disclosed. Public statements must be objective.
- Procedures should be established and followed for reporting irregularities and conflicts of interest. Requirements by clients for the professional to accept instructions which are perceived to be against the public interest must not be accepted.

The conduct of the professional requires self-regulation beyond that which is prescribed by legal restrictions and requirements. The degree and nature of such self-regulation is embodied in the professional codes, but leaves it to the professional to use their personal qualities to interpret and inform appropriate responses to particular situations. It is neither possible nor advisable to be prescriptive about all the details of professional practice.

The professional person must:

- be fully trained and broadly educated, with an understanding of the context within which decisions are made, as well as of their technical soundness
- ensure that they maintain competence by continually updating and extending their understanding of technical and professional developments
- contribute to the education and training of others, both during the formation period and throughout their professional development.

Interestingly, there has been no significant increase in the number of cases coming up for consideration since the new Rules of Practice were promulgated. About 20 to 30 cases are handled each year, usually concerning the smaller single-practitioner practices and inexperienced clients. Members occasionally seek advice from the Institution, but there are usually only about a dozen such references annually. The most frequent topic raised is possible conflict of interest. Of course, professional codes of practice need continuous review to ensure compatibility with contemporary factors, changing work patterns and changing legislation.

Professional values in practice

The brief case studies provided below illustrate the kinds of situations that can frequently arise on civil engineering projects, the values involved and the ways that decisions were/should be taken. In the case of the Lesotho project, a consultative system was created specifically for the project since no formal system was in place. In the case of the Channel Tunnel, the long-evolved and established system of approval by Parliament, representing the interests of the community with its system of public select committees, served this purpose. In both cases, time was set aside purely for the consideration of social and environmental issues.

The Lesotho Highlands water project

This project provides an interesting example of the methods by which the environmental and social aspects of a major project can, and should, be included in the project management arrangements of a major programme of construction works.

The Lesotho Highlands Region covers one-third of the area of the kingdom of Lesotho. This small country is completely surrounded by the Republic of South Africa. The Region is the source of the Senqu/Orange river, the largest and longest river in the area. The kingdom of Lesotho is poor and relatively undeveloped.

The primary objectives of the Lesotho Highlands Region project were:

- to redirect some of the water which presently flows out of Lesotho northwards towards the population centres of the Republic of South Africa
- to generate hydroelectric power in Lesotho using the redirected flows
- to provide regional social and economic development, water supply and irrigation in Lesotho.

These objectives were achieved by means of the construction of a series of dams, tunnels, pumping stations and hydroelectric works. Lesotho also benefits from the additional development of new roads, telecommunications, health clinics, community-based rural development projects and tourism. The total value of the projects in the Lesotho Highlands Region is in excess of £2 billion.

Such projects can bring disadvantages as well as benefits. Inundating land would displace local communities. An influx of foreign workers and job seekers could damage local culture and traditions and there are the negative effects of other environmental and social impacts. It was recognised that the positive benefits would outweigh the drawbacks and provisions only if it was stipulated that the standard of living of the affected population should not be inferior to that existing previously. Social and environmental considerations were highlighted and given prominence in the management structure of the project. The Lesotho Highlands Development Agency (LHDA) was formed to act as the owner of the project. The Agency then engaged engineers and contractors and co-ordinated the project with government ministries and public corporations.

No specific national environmental guidelines or procedures were in operation in Lesotho prior to the start of this project. The LHDA therefore adopted guidelines and detailed environmental specifications from other countries and international agencies. A series of social and environmental studies were commissioned and an environmental action plan concerning the impact on all aspects of local society developed.

The Channel Tunnel

The Channel Tunnel project cost about £9000 million. It took nearly seven years to construct and generated about 250 000 man-years of work. The area affected by it occupies about 500 acres of land in East Kent and a slightly greater area in France. The project required a high degree of international co-operation to ensure its completion. It provides a good illustration of how conflicts with public and external private interests can be reduced by formal consultation and deliberation.

The social consequences of the project in East Kent were considerable. Apart from the influx of construction workers, a large number of additional secondary jobs were generated. The existing social services had to be reviewed to ensure that they adjusted to the changing pattern of work and traffic in the area. All these factors were taken into account in the deliberations of the parliamentary committee conducting the public investigation into the consequences of the project.

Attention also had to be paid to the environmental implications and provision had to be made to ameliorate the effects of the development as far as possible. In the UK there are specially dedicated areas environmentally categorised as being of 'high landscape value', or of 'high nature conservancy value', or of 'special scientific interest'. The Folkestone terminal site encroached upon such areas. It was, therefore, important to identify the special features of the site.

During the select committee procedure, consideration was given to the conflicting interests involved, not only by the Committee itself but also by the petitioners and the experts. The maintenance of a balance between the legislators, the promoters of the scheme, the experts and the petitioners is of particular interest to the professional engineer who may be called as an expert.

It is possible to sum up the interests of the various parties briefly as follows:

- The promoters have the commercial interests of the private investors in mind, and also those of government policy as expressed through the sponsoring department.

- Parliament has in mind the best interests of the nation as a whole, as seen through the policies of the several political parties. It also cares for the individual rights of the electorate.
- The petitioners have in mind their own self-interest, or the interest of their particular organisation.
- The professional experts, including engineers, have in mind the factual aspects of the project, and the likely consequences of such developments on areas within their professional competence. It is particularly important that they give their advice impartially, competently, responsibly and independently, with proper professional integrity and discretion.

The procedures involved in evaluating the projects described above may seem to be elaborate and overbureaucratic. However, a systematic approach to conflict reduces the effect of personal biases and opinions. It thus contributes to the maintenance of goodwill and trust in society, and to the quality of professional advice available to the community.

Conclusion

The relationship between the values we profess as individuals, and the values developed and maintained by those of us responsible for giving informed and sound advice in our professional roles in a complex society, is not always easy to discern or manage. Engineers have a key role to play in society and their activities can have long-lasting and far-reaching effects. The stakes are therefore high as they seek to act in the highest traditions of their profession in providing objective and beneficial service not only to clients but to society at large. The role of the professional body as a means of prescribing, defining and promoting professional values and ethics, particularly through rules of practice, is crucial in ensuring the possibility of 'virtuous' practice on the part of individual engineers. This is important if members of the public are to continue to trust and value the skills and advice of professional engineers, both individually and corporately. In this chapter, we have seen how one professional body – the ICE and its members – has attempted to conceptualise and promulgate ethically responsible behaviour and reasonably objective advice-giving in the context of complex social and professional values and activities that often elude a simple analysis.

Institution of Civil Engineers: summary of rules of conduct

1 A member shall discharge their professional responsibilities with integrity and shall not undertake work in areas in which the member is not competent to practise.

2 A member shall uphold the dignity, respect and trustworthiness of the profession at all times.

3 A member shall have full regard for the public interest, particularly in relation to the environment and to matters of health and safety.

4 A member must understand and comply with the laws of the countries within which the member practises and with international law. Where professional codes of conduct exist in the countries concerned, a member should follow them. Where neither laws nor codes exist then a member should follow the Institution Rules of Professional Conduct.

5 A member, without disclosing the fact to the employer in writing, shall not be a director of, nor have a substantial interest in, nor be an agent for any company, firm or person carrying out any contracting, consulting or manufacturing business which is, or may be involved in, the work to which the employment relates. A member shall not receive, directly or indirectly, any royalty, gratuity or commission on any article or process used in or for the purposes of the work in respect of which the member is employed unless or until such royalty, gratuity or commission has been authorised in writing by the employer or client.

6 A member shall afford such assistance as may be reasonably given to further the education and training of candidates for the profession.

7 A member, either individually or through the member's organisation as an employer, shall afford such assistance as may be necessary to further the continuing professional development of the individual and of other members and prospective members of the profession in accordance with the recommendations made by the Council from time to time.

8 A member shall not maliciously or recklessly injure or attempt to injure, whether directly or indirectly, the professional reputation, prospects or business of another person.

9 A member who shall be convicted by a competent tribunal of a criminal offence, which in the opinion of the disciplinary body renders them unfit to be a member, shall be deemed to have been guilty of improper conduct.

10 A member shall not, in any manner derogatory to the dignity of the profession, advertise or write articles for publication, nor shall authority be given for such advertisements to be written or published by any other person.

11 A member shall, consistent with safety and other aspects of the public interest, endeavour to deliver to the employer or client cost-effective solutions. A member shall not comply with any instruction requiring dishonest action or the disregard of established norms of safety in design and construction.

12 A member shall discharge duties to the employer and the client both impartially and with complete fidelity. A member shall not receive any benefit or advantage relating to the work unless authorised by the employer or client

in writing. A member shall also declare any pecuniary interest in any other organisation involved with the work that is being undertaken for the employer and the client. Such a declaration may be made at the outset of the engagement or at any time when such a situation may become apparent during the progressing of the work for the employer or client.

13 A member shall not be the medium of payments made on the client's behalf unless so instructed by the client or employer; nor shall the member, in connection with work on which employed, place contracts or orders except with the authority of, and on behalf of, the client or of the employer as appropriate.

14 A member shall not improperly canvass or solicit professional employment, nor offer to make by way of commission or otherwise payment for the introduction of such employment unless disclosed to the employer.

15 A member shall not, directly or indirectly, attempt to supplant another engineer.

16 If requested to comment on another engineer's work, a member shall act with integrity and, except for routine or statutory checks or when the member's client or employer requires confidentiality, the member should advise the other engineer of their involvement.

PART IV

Values in education and training

Introduction

Traditionally, one of the main reasons for articulating professional values has been to influence and socialise new recruits. This theme has been illustrated in the discussion about artists (Chapter 3), clergy (Chapter 4) and social workers (Chapter 7). In the previous section, too, it was noted how the leaders of occupational groups employ codes of practice, conduct and ethics for this purpose.

For aspiring professionals, the gateway to membership has often been through higher education. This almost always involves taking a university degree, which might then be followed by more strictly vocationally oriented training. The newer, less well-established occupations have usually seen the introduction of degrees (as opposed to diplomas and certificates) as an important stage in achieving professional status and recognition. This has been the route adopted by many of the paramedical occupations, and those planning to become, for example, accountants and managers.

It is therefore appropriate that the next two chapters have been written by authors who have been heavily involved in university teaching, with experience of different countries and departments. As 'insiders', they are in a unique position to reflect on aspects of the current value socialisation process for their particular profession and its implications, not only for the students but also for those teaching them. In this connection, it should be noted that higher education itself employs a very large number of professionals and that academic institutions, with their associated values, are the work setting for many people.

The following two chapters complement each other well. They focus, respectively, on the values inherent in the formal curriculum, and those associated with a 'hidden curriculum' to which the students are exposed during work experience. Some may find these accounts disturbing. They certainly provide much food for thought about the implicit values conveyed to students by formal teaching processes and also by the more informal interaction with teachers and senior members of the profession in practice situations.

In Chapter 10 'Exploring values in legal education: an insider perspective', Eileen Fegan, an academic lawyer writing from a feminist viewpoint, takes a critical look at the values underpinning the curriculum in undergraduate legal education in universities. Drawing on research into legal education in the USA and the UK, she questions the nature of the values that are implicitly and explicitly imparted to students. Fegan questions the assumption that many law schools make that they should determine their curricula on the basis that all students will necessarily become practising professional lawyers. She suggests that they should adopt a more educational and critical approach which would encourage the study of 'law in context'. In her view, such an approach, more in keeping with the academic concept of a liberal arts degree, encourages students to question and explore the implications of traditional values and practices for themselves, rather than simply accepting them as given.

Fegan claims that the traditional legal curriculum, with its emphasis on the importance of private law and the value of a certain kind of objectivity, reflects and reinforces the hierarchical structure of the legal profession (largely white, male and middle class) and contributes to a failure to produce critical graduates or practitioners who are aware of biases and the wider social context and responsibilities surrounding law.

Having first made the case for a much closer examination of the implicit values underpinning the current system of legal education in the UK, Fegan outlines an approach that specifically sets out to give students permission to explore values and encourage a greater awareness of these issues. Fegan draws heavily on the work of Patricia Williams, a black feminist lawyer in the US. She describes how she has used Williams' writings to get students to 'think for themselves', develop their own approach, and record and reflect on their reactions. Fegan concludes that a great deal more needs to be done to open up the debate about what exactly a legal education is for amongst students, teachers, legal practitioners and members of the general public.

In Chapter 11 'Values, working lives and professional socialisation in planning', Huw Thomas, a town planner with considerable experience in practice and as a university teacher, focuses on the crucial first experience of the work placement for planning students. He shows how their reactions to a year-long placement might give some clues as to why the important professional value of commitment to equal opportunities, promoted by the professional body, the Royal Town Planning Institute, is rarely implemented or given much importance by local planning departments.

Drawing on his own research and the feedback from cohorts of students, Thomas speculates on the formative influence of the culture of the planning office on the student who is eager to fit in and learn 'the way we do things around here'. Many students contrast the education they have received while at university unfavourably with this first experience of professional practice. Some even go so far as to say they have not been prepared properly for practice. They place greater value on the 'active learning' on the job and the input from practising professional planners than on the more theoretical and 'passive learning' provided by the university.

In his fascinating analysis of the occupational culture of planners, Thomas stresses the tendency towards a stereotypical macho culture, the feeling of being embattled and misunderstood by outsiders, and the need for all 'to stick together' in the face of pressure from a number of stakeholders interested in their planning decisions. He argues that this explains the need to initiate the new recruit very quickly into the correct procedures and teach them the approved strategies and practical values for dealing with the outside world. Planning departments are an arm of local government and subject to the pressures found in these public sector environments. Thomas specifically makes a comparison with the similar attitudes towards colleagues reported among social workers and the importance attached in both settings to learning to fit in and 'not rocking the boat'. Finally, he analyses exactly why this type of work culture, with its own strong implicit and enacted values, is so inimical to the issues surrounding equal opportunities being promoted by the professional body and taught in the university.

Both of these chapters raise serious issues for reflection. The theory–practice gap is a constant theme in much of the literature on professional socialisation, particularly in the health field (Allen 2000; Bligh 2001; Grimshaw *et al.* 2002; Corlett *et al.* 2003; Sassi 2003). This is often coupled with the theme of disillusionment associated with student progress through training (Becker *et al.* 1961; Sinclair 1997).The student attitudes towards their university teaching reported by Thomas and Fegan pose the question: what exactly is the purpose of practitioner education in a university context? Is it to receive a liberal education or to produce a competent practitioner? Such a question also, of course, raises broader issues of what is the role of the university in modern society? What happens when there is a conflict between the academic values of those involved in teaching new recruits and practising professionals' perceptions of what are the most relevant and important things for the novice to learn in order to be a potentially useful future colleague?

The teachers, or some at least, may feel that university students should be encouraged to think, question received wisdom and challenge what they are being told or expected to do. In other words, students should cultivate the capacity to be reflective, lifelong learners with a well-developed critical sense so that they are able to evaluate their own practice and research and that of others. This would be in accord with the academic values traditionally espoused in higher education.

However, not surprisingly perhaps, many of the students described in these chapters appear to want simply to be taught the behaviours, 'rules' and 'facts' that will enable them to obtain the credentials and credibility needed to practise their chosen profession. 'Questioning' and the revelation of uncertainty, ambiguity and complexity is not welcomed or valued; it may simply increase levels of anxiety. This links back to their expectations of training and education and the nature of the tasks they perceive themselves as preparing to undertake.

Both chapters clearly illustrate the importance that students attach to direct experience of the work situation and observation and imitation of the way practitioners actually behave in the 'real world'. After all, it is the practising professionals who are actually carrying out the core tasks which identify the occupation as unique. The 'hidden curriculum' is a significant concept for understanding student attitudes and expectations here. It is important to recognise that it is not only what is formally taught and enshrined in the published curriculum that shapes student perspectives.

The rich literature on the socialisation of doctors and nurses provides many examples of the ways in which teachers and mentors inculcate their own values and the students attempt to make sense of what they need to learn in order to cope with an ever-growing mass of facts and tests of their grasp of this knowledge. In this context, the throwaway remark of a senior staff member, the feedback from other students slightly ahead of the novice's own group who reveal what it is 'really all about', and the way that practitioners in the work placement treat and talk about clients and colleagues when the novice is on placement may all be more significant in the development of values than those which are cognitively and formally imparted. It is this type of information that provides novices with the clues to constructing what is *really valued* in a particular setting, as distinct from what senior teachers and practitioners say *should* happen or what written codes *promulgate* as formal values and standards.

The issues raised here bring into sharp focus the clash that can occur between articulated formal, ideal professional standards, such as those found in professional codes and training curricula, and the enacted informal values that are actually to be found in everyday professional life. There is still a long way to go before the educational values of the academy and professional bodies and the values to be found in practice are brought together in a useful way for students, to enable them to become realistic, informed managers and critics of their own professional values. The fact that there is still a yawning gap between theory and practice, ideal and reality, classroom and office is an indictment of both the academic and professional spheres. Developments need to occur which allow students to become realistic reflective practitioners of professional values who can steer a steady course between what is theoretically prescribed and what is experienced in practice.

CHAPTER 10

Exploring values in legal education: an insider perspective

Eileen V Fegan

Introduction

This book addresses the need for a new understanding of professional values. In respect of the legal profession, values of justice, impartiality and objectivity are easily assumed and taken for granted by all players – the public, the judiciary, lawyers and, not least, by law students. In this chapter I explore from an experiential or 'insider' perspective the values embedded and mostly hidden within current models of legal education at university (i.e. non- vocational) level in the United Kingdom (UK).

The exploration will take place at various levels – the content of law school curricula, methods of teaching and assumptions about what constitutes a 'good' lawyer. My analysis will be permeated with an awareness of the power relations and the gender dimensions inherent in the value choices made in the 'intensely political' culture of the law school (Kennedy 1982: 40). I will explore how the content and conduct of legal education is productive of a 'masculinist' (Collier 1991) or macho culture. This operates effectively (and efficiently) as 'training' for both the legal profession and the hierarchical social world. It is within this culture that 'legal values' are defined and performed.

Assimilation to legal culture

By legal 'culture' I mean that blend of assumptions, attitudes and beliefs which defines law as unchangeable and unchallengeable. This culture structures legal education in ways averse to 'outsiders'. Rationality, relevance, impartiality and intellectual rigour are assumed essential in advocates and judges. These qualities have been criticised as partial, subjective and gender-specific because they are imbued with the behavioural norms traditionally associated with, and still expected of, men (Finley 1993). Upon entering law school, students are automatically aware of the superiority attached to these norms and traits. This superiority is reflected in, and reinforced through, the literature usually listed as essential first-year reading.

When I went to law school, *Learning the Law* by Glanville Williams was promoted as the law students' 'bible'. We were advised to turn frequently to it for 'helpful tips' such as '[m]en cannot improve the beauty of their countenances, but almost all of us can, if we wish, add to the attractiveness of our speech' (Williams 1982: 166). Williams also gave information about succeeding as a lawyer: 'women and non-whites are likely to experience particular difficulty [in securing a place at Bar Chambers]'. His response to this exclusion (like his grooming advice) emphasises the conditions of acceptance into legal culture: 'you should think long and hard before deciding to join the unhappy throng' (Williams 1982: 185). This raises fundamental questions about the responsibility of law schools for the qualities, and thereby the values, they seek to promote.

In law school, students are invariably taught how to be 'good' judges and 'good' lawyers. They are not required to question *what* is 'good' about lawyers' assumed qualities, or to develop awareness of the wider social, moral, political, cultural or economic effects of their practices. It has even been suggested by one critic that law schools are now firmly committed to teaching students how to be good capitalists (Ireland 2002). They promote economic efficiency arguments and the profit motive as the objective standard against which law's operation can be measured. Students and teachers should at least be aware of criticisms like this. Mostly, they are not.

There is a tremendous responsibility involved in teaching students to use a tool with the social power of law. Values are central to the work law students will eventually do, and the way in which they will do it. Consciously or not, they *will* contribute to the development of the society, whatever their eventual choice of work.

The power of lawyers to shape individual behaviour and social change is becoming more evident as law impinges further and deeper in many fundamental areas of life. Genetics and the new reproductive technologies are one example of an important new arena for legal endeavour. On a wider scale, the possibility of members of traditionally disempowered groups using human rights law to redress historic, systemic discrimination has been accentuated with the introduction of the Human Rights Act to the UK in 1998 (effective from October 2000). The corresponding growth of undergraduate courses and postgraduate degrees in human rights goes some way to redressing the historical focus of most law schools upon private law and commercial interests. However, the methods by which even the most obvious value-oriented subjects are taught can undermine any progress that might appear to have been made.

In this chapter I want to contribute to a new discourse on professional values. I will do this by seeking to raise awareness of law schools' and individual law teachers' roles in these processes. How might the schools and we, the teachers, best execute our inescapable responsibility for shaping and passing on the values of legal education directly for the benefit of students and indirectly for the good of society as a whole?

Exploring values in the law school curriculum

The aims of legal education may appear self-evident to observers. Certainly my experience is that many law students at entry level begin with an unquestioned certainty about what they are there to learn. Where does this certainty about the role and values of legal education come from? What role does the law school itself have in promoting the idea that 'I am not here to think, I am here to learn the law, get a good job and earn lots of money'?

There is a variety of motives for choosing law as a degree. However, broadly speaking, students who demonstrate any explicit motivation can be divided into two camps: those committed to 'social transformation' and those seeking 'social mobility'. Movement between the groups is always possible, more likely from the former to the latter. It is the latter group which is the main focus here.

My shorthand description, 'the social mobility student', reflects the widespread *initial* first-year response to the idea that there might be a variety of perspectives on law and that law itself might be the product of subjective values. It is based on nine years' experience (in four very different institutions) of challenging students to ask themselves why they are in law school and what they expect from a law degree. This challenge is a precursor to inviting students to set aside *all* expectations and embark upon an engaged and self-conscious learning experience. The end results of the process of value and assumption exploration are, of course, unpredictable. However, this value-sensitive approach has encouraged several initially hostile students to explore unanticipated ideas, issues and careers and to gain confidence in the process. This is one indicator of a worthwhile legal education where critical thought is nurtured. It is where I myself began to unravel the values of legal education through the methodology of my own insider, necessarily gendered, perspective. On my own journey I have been assisted by such students and by the work of other academics – in particular, earlier United States scholars who initiated the movement to situate law in its social and political context (Unger 1986).

The rise of 'critical legal studies'

In the 1980s, the 'Critical Legal Studies' movement gave rise to the exploration of legal education itself as a site of research, theoretical analysis and strategic engagement. The pioneer of this approach, Harvard Law Professor Duncan Kennedy, criticised the 'trade-school mentality' of many American law schools in their (metaphorical) 'attention to trees at the expense of forests'. He saw this as nonsense, but 'nonsense with a tilt ... [being] biased and motivated rather than random error' (Kennedy 1982: 40). His argument, that it is not the purpose or inevitable role of law schools to produce practising lawyers, has since gained currency in the UK, effectively dismantling the long-held perception of the law degree (or means of selecting its content) as objective, or value-free.

Several UK institutions have embraced the critical, 'law in context' approach, namely, Kent, Keele, Warwick, Lancaster, Birkbeck and, to a lesser extent, Cardiff (Thomson 1987). Others have been slow to reflect it in their programmes. They have remained dedicated to serving the narrowly defined needs of the profession. To this end the 'bread and butter' practitioner subjects – contract, trusts, torts, land and criminal law – are designated 'core' and taught in a formal way. According to this 'black-letter' tradition:

> Although law may appear to be irrational, chaotic and particularistic, if one digs deep enough and knows what one is looking for, then it will soon become evident that the law is an internally coherent and unified body of rules.
>
> (Sugarman 1991: 34)

Working on this kind of inward-looking, conservative assumption has established a model of British legal education that has proved very difficult to modify.

Some help was, however, forthcoming in the mid 1990s. The Lord Chancellor's Advisory Committee on Legal Education and Conduct (ACLEC) conducted a major review of legal education during this period and published its first consultation paper in 1996. This defined university teaching of law as 'a liberal arts degree' that should engender understanding of law in its social, moral, economic, political and cultural context. 'Core subjects' were replaced with 'foundations of legal knowledge' in a move to reflect the new contextual approach (ACLEC 1996: Appendix D). Yet, the term 'foundation' indicates that something essential, authentic and objective is being represented. A contrast is implied with that which is peripheral or unnecessary to learning the law. It suggests 'fully constituted subjects, clearly recognisable, describable, integrated and defined', whereas in fact, 'behind the seeming certainty of the presentation of these foundational elements lies a great deal of contention about the groupings, nomenclature and the actual topics selected for study' (Bottomley 1996: 3).

For Bottomley, critical scholars can take comfort in the difficulty of professional bodies in defining the foundational subjects and take advantage of this disagreement to expose them as merely 'heuristic devices'. The selection of particular subject areas as encapsulating *the* purpose of legal education is (always) value-laden. This becomes a problem when there is no recognition or acknowledgement of what these values are.

Current legal values

So what are the values that the current foundations of legal knowledge represent? Despite the addition of 'key elements and general principles of public law (including human rights) and the law of the European Union' (Bar Council and the Law Society *Joint Statement on Qualifying Law Degrees* 1999: Schedule 2), the emphasis on contract, property, land, trusts and torts still tips the balance in favour of private law, which regulates relations between private parties. This concentration of private law subjects mirrors and reinforces the supreme value attached to private interests and property in law and the legal profession. It reflects the influence of the propertied and upper classes upon the development of law and legal concepts in British legal history.

The roles, duties and responsibilities co-existing between the individual and the state are defined and policed by public law areas, i.e. criminal and constitutional and administrative law. There are also other highly relevant public law subjects, such as public international law that regulates relations between states and the use of force. Although these are now included in the 'general principles' promoted by ACLEC (1996: 21, 44, 51), these topics are not generally given such substantive treatment and are left to the 'optional' elements of the degree. In substantive terms, only constitutional and criminal law are represented as essential public law knowledge needed to satisfy the requirements of a 'qualifying law degree', which allows graduates to proceed to a one-year vocational training course without further examination.

Values and the structure of the profession

The composition of the judiciary and legal profession at the highest levels in the UK still reflects dominant interests and values, despite recent indicators suggesting greater potential for increased representation. Since 1988 more women than men have graduated in law. Female students get increasingly better results and have more success in gaining professional training contracts. Yet it was not until 2003 that the first female judge was appointed to the House of Lords and, at the start of the new millennium, the women sitting in the Court of Appeal and High Court constituted only 5.6% of the membership of the bench at the higher level, and only 14.3% in total (Cole 2000: 60).

In terms of age, sex, class, race and education, the judiciary has been described as a homogeneous group with 'a unifying attitude of mind, a political position, which is primarily concerned to protect and conserve certain values and institutions' (Griffith 1997: 7). In the face of these glaring indications as to the partiality of legal institutions, law continues to be represented by judges, professional bodies and the law school curriculum as a set of objective values to which *everyone* aspires.

Feminist scholars have argued that the greater the need to promote and defend the objective content of the law degree, the more specifically value-laden it may be found to be upon critical and contextual analysis (Bottomley 1996). Perhaps this is why such investigation is largely discouraged in the definition and teaching of the core/foundational subjects. Even where ostensibly theoretical courses are a compulsory element of the degree, as historically in Oxford and at Queen's University, Belfast, there is no guarantee that legal values will be examined.

Jurisprudence is traditionally understood as the philosophy of law. However, it is more often treated as an exposé of the grand theorists (notably all white males) on the *nature* of law, than as an opportunity to explore the *meaning* of law and the diverse subjects it is supposed to represent. While there is a body of jurisprudential literature written by critical theorists of race, gender, class and sexuality (Berns 1993), these analyses still have to make their way into most compulsory syllabi. While law at the highest level – the decision makers and the 'great thinkers' – continues to be represented by a white, male, middle class, Oxbridge norm, there is an urgent need to interrogate its values through legal education. At present, however, the standard curriculum remains at worst hostile and at best resilient to the influence of 'outsiders'.

Is there any justification for the present content of legal education?

The law degree is only the first or 'initial' stage in the four-stage structure of preparation for legal practice. This is followed by vocational study through the Legal Practice or Bar Vocational course. After this, there is a two-year training contract for solicitors and a one-year pupillage for barristers. Thereafter practitioners must engage in continuing professional education. There is, therefore, no necessity for rigidity among law school staff and students about what the curriculum should contain or how it should be taught.

Aspirant practitioners could learn much of the 'black-letter law' they need after their first law degrees. However, there is an unquestioned belief that there simply *are* certain subjects that fundamentally constitute the discipline and distinguish law from other areas of university study. This belief still influences the degree content, structure and, more pervasively, the methods by which it is taught. It permeates most law schools' external promotional literature and internal discussion of their decisions about the curriculum.

All students are encouraged to take those qualifying subjects now designated elective to the degree 'to keep their options open'. Thus, the assumption that anyone who has achieved the superior rigour demanded of a law
graduate would want to 'use it', still dictates the subjects offered and studied
in most law schools. This is unnecessary and unhelpful both to students'
intellectual progression and personal development as well as to their future
careers within the legal profession. They are limited too early from thinking
creatively, imaginatively and outside the boxes neatly drawn for them in
law school.

Consider, for example, the reaction of one of my law school contempor-
aries (now a successful partner in private practice) when I asked about her
experience with test cases in which lawyers attempt to expand the current
boundaries of law to the benefit of their client. She was aghast: 'I wouldn't
know where to start ... I basically just fill in forms and follow the procedure'
was the gist of her reply.

There is no justification for maintaining, as many law schools and individual teachers still do, that their purpose is to teach students how to 'think
like a lawyer'. As a former student (and now fellow academic) commented
in response to the almost constant focus on legal method, 'a law degree is
a life sentence! '(Rackley 1997). Three years of sidelining students into dry,
technical and inaccessible legal subjects, discouraging them from considering the bigger, social picture and orienting them to find the 'right
answer' to any problem, can have a lifelong effect on their ability to think
about law in anything other than abstract, absolutist, or black and white
terms. This mode of thinking, understood as 'legal reasoning or method',
can condition, and may even reconstitute, the personality of the 'successful'
law student.

What are we teaching law students to do?

Legal method is that process by which students learn, and lawyers or judges
'do' law. It is the process of detached, abstract and neutral application of
rules to facts. It has been defined as:

> The hypostatization of exclusive categories and definitional polari-
> ties ... the existence of transcendent, acontextual, universal legal
> truths or pure procedures ... the existence of objective
> 'unmediated' voices by which those truths find their expression.
>
> (Williams 1991: 8–9)

The prioritisation of the acquisition of this approach in legal education as an
objective, value-free method of resolving legal disputes serves to obscure the
range of choices available in deciding any particular case. Encouraging
students to see the choices of adjudicators as neutral and impartial is unsatisfactory. It is problematic from a critical values perspective.

Furthermore, the importance of inculcating this skill, considered widely to be the *raison d'être* of legal education, is invoked to justify the very subjective choices that are actually made when law schools decide *how* to teach the foundational subjects. Implicit in reproducing this uncritical and unself-conscious choosing of certain values over other existing and possible values (in making proficiency in legal method a condition of the law degree) is the aim of reproducing this very hierarchy. A similar hierarchical culture permeates the law school.

It would be more ethical and honest to acknowledge that these choices represent dominant perspectives, namely, those of the judges who have the power to implement their values, albeit backed by the authority of law. Feminist critics, in particular, have made the observation that since judges are predominantly male, white, and middle or upper-middle class, their judgements most often reflect the prejudices shared by this group of people (Finley 1993). 'Legal method' is used to justify the very subjective choices that are actually made when legal reasoning takes place. Yet, the obfuscation of perspective is inculcated in law students as simply '*the* way to do law' through continued reinforcement of the importance of this art in traditional legal education.

An alternative approach: an experiential search for values

So far, I have stressed the way in which even the most value-oriented subjects in law such as jurisprudence are taught can still undermine any progress that might appear to have been made in altering the overall trends in legal education and making it more sensitive to an awareness of values – its own and others.

I will now examine the potential offered by an experience-based methodology for injecting into legal education an awareness of, and a commitment to, exploring values. This methodology is inspired by the work of American feminist and critical race scholar, Patricia Williams.

In her highly acclaimed *Alchemy of Race and Rights*, Williams discusses how law, though aspiring to profound goals such as justice, fairness and equality, often fails those most in need of its protection (Williams 1991). Relying upon her own experience as a black woman and commercial lawyer, she examines the values inherent in Anglo-American legal concepts, language, reasoning and methods, including those of traditional legal education. The relevance of her approach to the issues raised in this chapter lies in the way that her material, and particularly the *style* in which it is presented, can be used to stir an awareness of legal values within law students.

I use her book as a tool to experiment with and engage students' assumptions and consciousness. It opens:

> Since subject is everything in my analysis of law, you deserve to
> know that it is a bad morning. I am very depressed. It usually
> starts with some random thought like 'I hate being a lawyer'.
> (Williams 1991: 1)

This can be quite unsettling for those who have just begun to think that
they have a grasp on their legal studies. For others it is liberating – 'I
didn't know I was allowed to think/write what I really think about law'. It
is difficult to convince most students (and indeed colleagues) of the method
in the seeming madness and chaos of letting subjective perspectives loose
on law. However, the practical benefits become evident with time and
persistence.

In my pre-final and final-year undergraduate courses, *Philosophy* and
Gender and Law, students are given the opportunity to devise their own
(100% assessment) essay title, reflecting whatever personal interest the
course may have engendered or touched upon. This freedom requires them
to be active in identifying and tracking the wider implications of *their own*,
as well as legal, values and to develop skills of independent research,
thought and confidence in their own ideas.

As a result of the success with those students, I now introduce first-years
to Williams' material in the compulsory foundational *Introduction to Law*
module. This is designed to develop and practise legal skills. I do this in a
deliberate attempt to catch their consciousness and encourage them to work
on their own awareness before it becomes 'set' by, and within, the confines
of legal tradition.

One student wrote to me saying that, while it was all very interesting,
first-years already have so much to read and master in this unfamiliar
subject that there is no time to waste on the personal gripes or ramblings of
the disaffected. My response was to encourage him to question further the
assumptions about what students 'have' to learn. He was given permission
and space within the course to dedicate time to non-traditional texts, to the
process of understanding his own and law's implicit values, and to become
aware of how legal values become almost imperceptibly ingrained through
the very use of dense, inaccessible texts and jargon. Contrary to his original
fears, he very quickly ceased to feel so intimidated by the 'seriousness' and
perceived authority of traditional legal texts. He read them faster and
became comfortable in criticising and commenting upon them.

Resistance, exemplified by this student's initial reaction, is to be expected
both from colleagues and students. Most chose law because they thought of
it as a definitive, closed and relatively 'safe' discipline, far removed from the
ambiguities of the social sciences or the humanities. New law students tend
to be conservative, protective of their own perceived intelligence, and
unlikely to trust non-traditional texts and methods. My approach has been
variously described (initially, at least) as 'irrelevant, airy-fairy and random'.
However, initial confusion and mistrust can be, and has been, overcome by
accepting it as natural, necessary and a short-lived precursor to reaching

the goal of empowering students to discover, examine and develop an individual and independent response to the values of law.

Much progress has already been made in diversifying UK legal literature as a consequence of similar ideas. Acknowledging that at a later stage 'it may well be too late to introduce the idea that the rules of the game are not neutral and that groups of people are likely to be differentially affected by the outcome', several scholars at Kent Law School developed a critical first-year text, in an effort to 'question commonsense assumptions (or authoritative pronouncements) about law and about the relationship between law and society, even before the student has begun to "think like a lawyer"' (Mansell *et al.* 1995: iii).

Experimenting with values

Patricia Williams' work directly challenges students' preconceptions of what it means to 'do' law in both substance and style. It is immediately effective in unsettling long-established and 'taken for granted' legal values. It is material to which they invariably react and is therefore a useful tool in getting (especially first-year) students to become aware of their own role in the education process. By asking them to record and reflect upon their reactions, I have enabled them to identify and assess their own position *vis-à-vis* law. This allows them to know from firsthand experience the inevitable impact of personal perspective upon the process of interpretation. In this, their study begins to mirror the role of judges in interpreting legal texts and developing the law.

In the application of this approach, I have given students the opportunity to adopt (and swap) 'insider' perspectives – including that of judge – in respect of both real and hypothetical cases. For example, first-year students are asked for a decision upon the facts of a 1992 case involving a pregnant woman who refused a medically recommended caesarean section on religious grounds. No precedent involving sufficiently similar facts exists, so unsuspecting first-years are able to experience firsthand the judicial phenomenon of making the law up as they go. It forces them to realise the effect of their own values and beliefs upon this supposedly 'objective' process – especially when they are exposed to the range of opinions among their classmates. The practical purpose of the experiment is not to change anyone's mind. It opens up law and legal reasoning to debate, enabling a self-conscious and responsible assessment of values.

Both Williams' experiential analyses and my own experimental teaching of law strike many legal academics and most lawyers as too anecdotal and irrelevant to influence either the elevated and 'universal' discourse or the 'practical' business of law. Yet, its ability to elicit an immediate, often unthinking, response provides a necessary litmus test of assumed values which are largely unquestioned and taken for granted in law and legal education. As one commentator notes, Patricia Williams' work:

offers receptive readers a means by which to turn their own sense of defensiveness outward toward what they know, and perhaps to imagine what they want the law and its context to resemble. For less sympathetic readers, Williams offers a challenge to some well-worn precepts and a chance to change their minds.

(Bruhl 1996: 2014)

Style as substance

It is, however, perhaps through her idiosyncratic methodology of writing about law 'in [her] own voice' that Williams has made the greatest contribution to a new discourse on legal values. Her narrative style 'challenge[s] the usual limits of [legal] discourse by using an intentionally double-voiced and relational, rather than a traditionally legal black-letter, vocabulary' (Williams 1991: 6). It has encouraged others, including me, to experiment with law teaching, research and assessment. Collectively, scholars writing within this narrative and critical genre have succeeded to a large extent in challenging and undoing the power of legal language and literature to overwhelm students and prevent 'outsiders' from participating in a debate about legal values.

Legal reasoning has been described by Harvard critical legal scholar, Martha Minow, as 'the practice of perceiving problems through categories and acceptance of the consequences assigned to particular legal categories' (Minow 1991: 1). It is often defended as law's only way to make sense of the immeasurable complexity of life and infinite combinations of factual situations. Yet, a deeper awareness of the reasons behind, and the effects of, law's particular forms of categorisation produces further insight into the values hidden by this 'practical' justification. Law's categories separate, divide and define the legal subject in terms of 'the individual', who is ultimately disempowered before the overwhelming power of law.

This is why feminists need 'to think laterally, in terms of relations, through and over categories' (Bottomley 1996: 4). Law's 'static, unyielding, totally uncompromising point of reference' (Williams 1991: 10) which warns outsiders to 'stay away' must rather be viewed as a call to redefine legal subjectivity in more potent and challenging terms, such as group interests. Those subjected to common social phenomena of racism and sexism, for instance, may still engage with the law. But they need to do this through methods which value their own experiences of what it feels like, first, to suffer denigration or abuse, and second, to have it denied or obliterated through the unseeing eyes of lawyers, judges and law teachers who, more often than not, 'capitulate so uncritically to a norm that refuses to allow for difference' (Williams 1991: 11).

Doing it differently

Williams' work demonstrates how, practically and theoretically, all legal categories may be examined from alternative perspectives. Simple questions that are largely overlooked in legal education, such as *who* defines 'relevance', 'reason' and 'objectivity' and *whose* experience is negated in the labeling of 'irrelevance', 'emotion' and 'subjectivity', can eventually lead to actual changes in both the substance and interpretation of law.

One concrete example of this is the success of feminist research into and analyses of the inherent subjectivity of supposedly objective legal standards such as 'reasonableness'. This concept has been opened to interpretation from a variety of perspectives (Conaghan 1996). Progress has also been achieved in demonstrating how the male perspective has been accepted and reinforced as 'the norm' in those cases where battered women who 'snapped' after years of abuse, killing their partners, tried to use the defence of provocation against a murder charge. Their actions would not fit into the common law definition of provocation as 'a sudden and temporary loss of self-control' because that had been developed by a male judiciary reflecting upon the experience of the jealous husband finding his wife with another man or the young man taunted about his sexual orientation or prowess.

As a result of concerted efforts by feminist scholars (including men such as Nicolson [1995]), women's support groups and practitioners, the effect upon the particular *individual* of the alleged provocation is now at least recognised in the interpretation of what constitutes a reasonable reaction. For the moment, however, the long-standing definition itself still stands.

Law graduates need to be aware of the vast element of subjectivity and choice available to judges in deciding cases, in interpreting and developing law, and to practitioners in constructing arguments around it. Such awareness will then promote greater responsibility for the social consequences of law's hidden values, as well as its divisive categories and practices. At present these are uniformly (though mostly inadvertently) replicated and reinforced in the teaching of the 'core' subjects and the 'standard' approach to developing legal skills. Students need to have the opportunity to look beneath the need for clarity, certainty and standardisation proclaimed by judges in cases and law teachers in textbooks before they, too, are repelled by the messiness of recognising human differences.

Williams argues that 'standards are nothing more than structured preferences' (1991: 103) of those already holding power. If this is so, it is unethical within legal education not to explore the values of substantive legal standards and the supposedly 'objective' legal methods used to justify the selection of certain preferences over others. This has practical consequences for law students' educational experiences and for their later perspective on the world once fully qualified. These standards reflect the differential treatment and positioning of non-preferred characteristics, ideals and values within the law school hierarchy itself, as well as the fear of losing out to them.

From conformity to collectivity

Unspoken value judgments about alternative (or non-foundational) areas of study and methods of teaching are made; these *devalue* those who seek to redress this ethical imbalance. Those who make these judgements do so in a manner mirroring supposedly neutral rules of evidence in the courtroom. The ever-present assumptions of what constitutes a 'serious' legal academic (and law student) reflect a gendered (male) and racial (white) prototype, leaving little scope for other interpretations. Yet, the message is conflicting.

When women display the behaviour and attitudes seen as 'assertive' and 'powerful' in male colleagues, they risk being constructed as 'difficult, problematic, not a team player'. This makes it difficult for women, together with non-white and non-traditionally identified men, to assess how to play the academic game. Some admittedly buy into this culture, perhaps because from any individual's perspective, it is safer than pushing the traditional boundaries on your own.

I have identified in various institutions a 'resigned conformity' (or battle weariness) of those women who having fought for change, but have found it ultimately futile or short-lived. Others, especially younger women, show a 'predisposed conformity' – believing, or declaring to believe, that there is simply no gender issue. This can be understood when both perspectives are considered from their own subject positions. Why should women who have worked so hard just to survive and get promoted in the law school continue to fight on behalf of newcomers who are ungrateful or even hostile to their efforts? For the latter, of course, there is a very real threat that they might not get (or stay) within the academy if they don't play by the 'rules'. Yet, if efforts are made by both to share experiences and understand each other's positions, new alliances can be forged and necessary relationships of trust and support can be built.

Research already conducted by Professors Clare McGlynn (1999) and Celia Wells (2002) into the work allocations of, and on the different gender identity types adopted by, female legal academics have sparked the development of formal organisations and informal networks, such as the national 'Women Law Professors Network'. As a model of collective awareness raising, reflection, engagement and resistance, similar institutional, local and regional groupings can both keep the values of the law school under scrutiny and inject legal education with much needed alternative perspectives.

Conclusion

This exploration of the curriculum, dominant pedagogy and culture of UK law schools from an insider perspective has identified certain core, conservative values. These are remarkably persistent, despite efforts by critical, feminist and 'outsider' legal scholars generally to revolutionise the law school experience with an awareness of alternative perspectives and values. Perhaps this is because this discourse has taken place only at the academic and largely theoretical level. It is, therefore, easily ignored by law teachers. They are happy, or more likely secure, with things remaining as they are.

A wider debate on values in legal education is needed that includes and engages those who have a vested belief in its objectivity. Questions as to what, how, and why we teach what we teach need to be discussed more generally, and not restricted to a few distinguished socio-legal journals and academic conferences.

Vocational trainers, practitioners and judges also need to be engaged in the debate about what law school is for. The classroom, assessment methods and criteria, and the research agenda – to name a few examples – need to be opened up to wider scrutiny, including that of students and non-law specialists. This may make law teachers uncomfortable as they become more vulnerable to an examination of their own professional and personal values by colleagues and students. Yet, to resist such a development in the interests of an easy life is unethical. It assumes that it is better to pretend to have or see no values other than those implicit in law itself. To stand ethically paralysed and personally silenced by the threat of a 'greater' power is hardly a legacy we would wish to pass to our graduates.

CHAPTER 11

Values, working lives and professional socialisation in planning

Huw Thomas

Introduction

This chapter examines the way values embed themselves within the working lives of professional town planners. It will tend to focus upon a particular key aspect of planning – the consideration of planning applications. I will explore some of the implications of the embedding of values in attempts to change professional values and attitudes. It draws on research projects into various aspects of professional life conducted over a number of years (though not with this chapter in mind), personal experience of professional practice and generally unsystematic discussions with students who have been on year-long professional placements as part of their studies at Cardiff University. (I should point out that both male and female students were involved in the discussions, but there were no minority ethnic students, nor disabled students.) The chapter consists of well-informed speculation rather than rigorous testing of a narrowly defined hypothesis, with the hope that it will stimulate discussion and, in time, more rigorous treatment of the topic.

The background to the discussion is the attempt by the Royal Town Planning Institute (RTPI) – since at least the early 1980s – to persuade its members to take the promotion of equal opportunities more seriously in their day-to-day work. There is scope for debate about how single-minded the Institute has been in trying to change the attitudes of professionals. But even if it is conceded that equal opportunities has never been its top priority, the Institute can still point to a series of initiatives relating to sexism, racism and promoting physical accessibility in the built environment. It has commissioned studies on ways of increasing the proportions of planners from black and ethnic minorities. It has also supported the work of two standing committees ('panels' in its organisational vocabulary) with a brief to oversee its activities on race and gender.

However, all the relevant evidence shows that planners do not regard the promotion of equal opportunities as an important part of their work; indeed, most planners barely understand what promoting equal opportunities means (Little 1994; Thomas 2000). It has been suggested that this gulf between the professional institute and its members reflects the sensitivity of working planners to local political priorities (Thomas 2000), central government policies and guidance (Loftman and Beazley 1998), and/or assumptions embedded in the legal system which frames all planning intervention (Lo Piccolo and Thomas 2001).

This chapter complements these discussions by considering how the idea of equal opportunities might find a place, or fail to do so, in the day-to-day routines of planners – routines which will be responsive to a number of factors, including, but perhaps going beyond, those just mentioned. The assumption underlying the discussion is that 'work experience is of central importance' in the development of workers' consciousness and understanding of the world (Dale 1976), and that central to what is explained is the experience of work itself.

Equal opportunities, professionals and their values

'Equal opportunities' has become jargon. It might be helpful to say a little about what it might mean and how it might relate to values of professionals. The term is interpreted in a number of ways, but there is an important distinction between a concern for fairness to *individuals* who are involved in certain processes and procedures (the focus for action is then ensuring that relevant criteria alone should influence their treatment) and a concern that a *certain pattern of outcomes for groups* be established (the focus for action becomes defining a just distribution and using appropriate mechanisms, e.g. quotas or a questioning of the very activity itself, to achieve it).

These perspectives are part of broader (political) understandings of how unfairness and injustice are generated. Putting the matter crudely, the former position sits easiest with a view of racism and sexism as inappropriate behaviour by particular individuals. The assumption is that, although individuals are socialised in certain ways, they can still be persuaded or coerced to change their behaviour; once this is done, then the problem is solved. The latter position sees discriminatory acts as manifestations of systematic injustices which shape the very way in which society is organised, the way people are brought up and educated, and so on. Rectifying the behaviour of individuals, or tinkering with procedures, is necessary but not sufficient for addressing this systemic injustice.

There has not been widespread discussion within the RTPI of the different conceptions of equal opportunities. It appears, however, that the first view is implicit in much of what the Institute has done – for example, advising planners on how to organise the translation of technical material. The implication being that procedures which assume fluency in English may put some citizens at an unfair disadvantage, but that once the procedure is improved then the demands of fairness will have been met. One might have thought that this kind of concern would be easily accommodated by professionals inasmuch as it is the less radical of the two approaches. However, I will suggest that in a somewhat unexpected way, it is this approach which may be the more difficult for planners to adopt as a good way to practise. I will suggest that resistance to a pretty thin conception of equal opportunities is best explained by reference to occupational cultures of planners, how they regard what they know and how they make sense of their working lives.

Acquiring knowledge in planning

In the UK, planning has been a graduate-entry profession for decades. That has not prevented a chasm developing between university education and professional practice. This is a relatively recent phenomenon. The divide has grown as university teaching of planning has come to be the preserve of career academics, with a concomitant sharp decline in involvement by practising planners. This pattern began in the late 1960s, and has become universal. The emphasis placed by universities on research activity and on the professionalising of university teaching (e.g. by the founding of the Institute of Learning and Teaching) has simply strengthened a trend that has been affecting the training of planners for many years (Thomas 1980).

The perceived theory–practice gap

A common view in professional practice – shared by many academics – is that there is a 'theory–practice gap' (Allmendinger 1998). One consequence of this is that the relevance of university education for professional practice can be questioned. One of the most common initial comments of students who have completed a 'sandwich' year in professional practice is that their university education did not prepare them properly for practice; the more truculent make it plain that they see it as having been 'irrelevant'.

It is tempting to dismiss these concerns as the fruit of profound philistinism, but I believe that to be misguided. A more persuasive explanation of these sentiments is that the very clear reorientation of university education towards academic norms of achievement and conduct has exposed an important feature of planners' professional culture – namely, the primacy accorded to experience rather than scholarly research, as a source of knowledge. It is likely that many, perhaps most, professions in the UK share this trait.

Direct experience versus university education

Sinclair traces the introduction and promotion of the idea in medical training that certain important kinds of knowledge can only be acquired through direct multi-sensory contact between the individual practitioner and an individual patient (Sinclair 1997). He argues that there remains a tension at the heart of medical training and practice between the respect accorded to direct individual experience and the importance of science (and the idea of knowledge as impersonal) as a basis for the status of the modern medical profession.

There is no equivalent study of planning, but there is plenty of anecdotal evidence of the respect accorded to practical experience. Moreover, in planning, the countervailing weight of science/scholarship is nothing like as great as that in the medical case. Planning's history and current practice is littered with public controversies which cannot be resolved by any kind of conclusive proof and, indeed, in some cases revolve around contested evidence, e.g. in relation to whether road-building increases or alleviates traffic congestion. I suggest that part of the attraction of experience is that it can appear to provide a basis for the confidence and certainty in judgement that is a mark of the competent planning professional. (Atkinson [1984] makes a similar point on clinical training for medical students being a training in dogmatism.)

The perceptions of undergraduate town planners

Reflecting upon a year in professional practice 'sandwiched' into their university degree, undergraduate planners emphasise how strange and new the first experience of entering the planning office was. It takes no prompting for some sharp distinctions to be drawn between what they were taught in their three years in university and what they learned in the office. 'Practical planning knowledge' is the phrase used by one student to describe what the year of experience taught her, as opposed to 'just being told' about things in the university.

Analytical distinctions (between policy areas, for example) which dominate the academic curriculum are compared unfavourably with the way they experience things as 'linked up' in their office placement. The university education is universally regarded as unsuitable. A typical comment is: 'We joined the planning course to become practical town planners.' It is by no means clear to student planners how a social science based university education helps them.

The contestability of theses in the social sciences must be a serious liability for those who are seeking practicality and certainty. In this view of what constitutes worthwhile knowledge, the existence of competing justifications for promoting equal opportunities already places a question mark over its status as professionally relevant knowledge. My experience of teaching a module on equal opportunities to planning students is that most enthuse about learning how to apply standards of accessibility when evaluating buildings. However, they are at best bored, and often made anxious, by the sometimes passionate arguments which arise around how disability should be defined, and the implications of different approaches to definitions for the promotion of equal opportunities.

Active learning on the job

A striking feature of student accounts of how they learn during their professional placement is how (selectively) active they are in the process. Students realise quite quickly that they must take initiatives to ensure that they can perform adequately in the office. For example, for all five students in one focus group, careful observation of more senior officers was an important way of learning skills, both mundane and sophisticated (e.g. answering the telephone in an appropriate way, or negotiation). However, other forms of active learning appeared to be beset by more anxiety – learning 'through necessity' was offered as a description by one person, and there were wry smiles of recognition as an anecdote was offered of a panic-filled afternoon searching through files for information for a senior officer.

In my experience, this approach to learning is considerably more active than the approach adopted by the same students in relation to their full-time university studies. I would speculate that this is a combination of the way lecturers present themselves (as experts, uniquely able to define the contours of a subject or specialism) and a view held by students of theoretical knowledge as something to be absorbed passively, prior to use in practice, its usefulness presumably varying directly with its degree of certainty (a perspective Sinclair [1997] found in trainee doctors). Engagement with, and questioning of, theory – an activity valued by academics – has no place in this view of knowledge and its acquisition.

In the practice setting, no less than in the university, active learning does not extend to questioning the knowledge being offered. One female student spoke of how key lessons had been taught by someone who 'sat me down, patted me on the head and told me'. (Many other students had identified a sympathetic individual in the office who would teach them important aspects of the job.) As the quotation implies, these relationships impart more than just technical information about planning – the manner of the teaching helps initiate the novice planner into a set of social relations through which planning is undertaken in that setting.

The importance of the culture of the work setting

When a group of students midway through a year-long placement discussed what they had learned so far, central to the session were variations on the theme of 'you have to know your office culture' (as one put it). Communicating with colleagues and people outside the office was part of this ('appreciating where everyone's coming from' said another). The student planner is learning to fit into a set of social relations which, inevitably, are power-laden, and very likely share at least some of the limitations and injustices associated with the wider social context. But questioning any perceived flaws – for example, by drawing attention to sexism or racism in the work-place – will threaten the delivery mechanism which is teaching the new planner how to do the job; moreover, as we will see in the next section, there are strong pressures on planners to stick together in the workplace.

'Under threat': the occupational context and culture of planners

In an account of social workers specialising in child care, Pithouse (1994) describes how a particular kind of colleagueship (his term) was forged which helped the workers 'construct their activities as orderly and credit-able' in an often hostile and uncertain environment. Planners, too, operate in an environment which can fairly be described as threatening, if not always actually hostile. Key characteristics are:

- Making plans and making decisions on planning applications creates benefits for some and costs, or losses, for others. Often there is a great deal at stake for individuals and groups. There are no reliable data about physical attacks on planners but they appear to occur pretty regularly, and there has been at least one fatal assault in the last ten years. One of the student planners admitted being threatened with death by a disgruntled member of the public, and many others recalled being intimidated by planning applicants or members of the public.
- There are very occasional rumours (and seemingly very few instances) of corruption, but an understandable public perception that planning could be corrupt (given the amounts of money to be made from favourable decisions).
- Formal responsibility for decisions rests with councillors, who become interested in scrutinising (and attempting to influence) planners' judgements. This comes as a shock to many student planners – one commented, 'I didn't connect planning and politics before' – which probably reflects how they wished to perceive planning, rather than what was actually in their curriculum or textbooks.
- There are a number of opportunities (defined by law) for members of the public to make representations to planners, and, subsequently, test planners' judgements.
- Testing of planners' judgements is still dominated by a judicial (and hence adversarial) approach – the majority of planners will have given

evidence as expert witnesses to some kind of public inquiry (and been cross-examined) at some time during their careers. Many experience this regularly. Being asked/allowed to present and defend a planning case, either by exchange of written submissions or in person at a hearing, is regarded as simultaneously traumatic and a great opportunity – a kind of 'rite of passage' – by student planners.

- The technical content of professional practice is not great and swathes of planning standards and guidelines are unsupported by research evidence. Monitoring and evaluation are rarely undertaken with any rigour (Reade 1987). All this leaves planners vulnerable when challenged.

Planning office culture

I suggest that some key factors have encouraged planners to develop an occupational culture which has features inimical to taking promoting equal opportunities seriously.

The first of these is *a dominant concern with process and procedure.* This provides a bulwark against accusations of partisanship, and also a very real protection against attempts on the part of less powerful interests to unduly influence planners' judgements. (In truth, very powerful interests often insist on being accommodated and leave it to the planners to work out how to ensure that the usual procedural niceties are observed).

Secondly, there is *a sense of sharing a beleaguered position, and of being open to unfair attack for mercenary and self-interested reasons.* Planners tend to develop either or both of the following reactions to the foibles of the public, councillors and developers: a righteous indignation or a blackish humour. The sentiments of American planners recorded by John Forester (1993) would be well understood by UK planners: 'If something goes wrong, the planners did it. If something goes right, the City Council members claim credit for it.' This sense of identity is strongest among those groups of planners most often and most directly in the firing line – namely, those dealing with planning applications (McLoughlin 1973) – but is also evident elsewhere. One student planner mid-way through a placement year in an economic development unit found the most surprising (and, he said, 'shocking') aspect of professional practice was that 'a load of slagging off goes on', which I would interpret as the development and consolidation of colleagueship through a defining of demonised 'others'.

These two features help explain a curious aspect of planning offices already referred to in this chapter, namely, the very great effort expended on teaching new entrants the procedures, processes and standards of their new office (Nicholson 1991). In a hostile world, new recruits have to be schooled in the ways of their office and taught to accept them; then they can contribute to, and benefit from, the atmosphere of (beleaguered) colleagueship. This is the experience of placement students – their major lessons are in

learning protocols of dealing with councillors, fellow officers, planning applicants and other members of the public – cf. Baum on a similar US experience (Baum 1997).

I would speculate that the greater the adversarial content of the work of a
group of planners, the more likely they are to inflect their colleagueship with
stereotypically masculine behaviour and attitudes. Whatever the accuracy of
the speculation, some planning offices certainly have very stereotypically
gendered behaviour. This has come out quite clearly in the experiences of
two female students who recently spent consecutive years in a development
control section where all the other professional staff were men. One was
accounted a great success by her colleagues and manager. She was unag-
gressively flirtatious, and presented an inability to plan her time and express
herself formally as an endearing dizziness. (It had earned her quite a poor
degree.) She was 'looked after'.

The second student did not wish to be looked after, but also rejected other
roles on offer, e.g. becoming 'one of the boys'. She had a stressful year,
feeling that she was not fully accepted as a colleague, that she might be let
down by co-workers and was not being encouraged to seek assistance from
her manager. Her practical and emotional support came from female
support workers – administrators and secretaries who seemed to regard the
gendered 'games' of the male planners with a mixture of exasperation and
contempt.

The gendered nature of planning life also emerged in accounts of conflict
with the public. For women, sexist abuse ('you old slag', and so on) was not
uncommon; one consequence was to emphasise gender roles within the
office, as (male) colleagues took care to 'protect' their womenfolk by antici-
pating visits and meetings which might be problematical.

Conclusion

A wealth of research evidence shows that promoting equal opportunities is
not regarded as important by professional planners. The particular concern
of this chapter has been why student planners who have undertaken, or are
in the midst of, work placements appear to find it difficult to say anything
about equal opportunities when discussing their experience of work, even
though they have only recently studied equal opportunities in university.
They seem to struggle to find a way of using the concepts and concerns
associated with the promotion of equal opportunities to make sense of their
work experiences. The students quoted above, who had so many vivid
things to say about their introduction to professional life, typically fell silent
when asked whether issues associated with equal opportunities arose in
their placements.

The possible inference of this discussion is that the values and concepts
associated with promoting equal opportunities struggle to find any kind of
purchase in the life of the professional planner – first, because planners

valorise experiential knowledge acquisition, and secondly, because the occupational culture of planners contains values and attributes inimical to the concerns of equal opportunities. The combination of these factors squeezes equal opportunities off the conceptual and normative map of novice planners as they struggle to come to terms with their introduction to practice.

Planners value knowledge that can guide (and justify) professional practice. This means that contestable social science will always appear a poor basis for practice compared to the apparent certainty and specificity of that which is directly experienced. For novice planners, the intellectual and normative contestability of equal opportunities immediately devalues it as knowledge for practice, and its absence from the concerns of existing, experienced practitioners – valued sources of applicable knowledge – confirms its marginality as a source of professional knowledge.

Equal opportunities does not figure in the instruction experienced planners impart to newcomers because planners have developed an occupational culture which emphasises the importance of procedural correctness (fine-tuned to suit local pressures and sensitivities), of neutrality and a studied impartiality, and of the need to constantly guard against (and protect each other against) hostile others motivated by self-interest. They are predisposed to be suspicious of a call to promote equal opportunities which demands changes to procedures (albeit changes which it is claimed are designed to secure fairness), which imply that individuals and/or groups have either been unfairly treated or might be so treated in the future, and casts a shadow over (stereotypically masculine) attitudes or behaviour which are culturally encoded as associated with standing up for oneself in the face of unfair criticism.

The concerns associated with promoting equal opportunities can appear to emanate from a very different kind of world to that in which planners operate. Planners know that which they experience – they *know* that procedures are applied impartially; they *know* that they are often the butt of unjust criticism and hostility; they *know* that the ideas and concerns associated with equal opportunities do not seem to make any better sense of these experiences than the occupational culture already in place.

If this analysis is reasonably accurate then the promotion of equal opportunities within planning may be made easier by:

- ameliorating the adversarial nature of the process
- reducing the pressure of scrutiny on planners by councillors
- limiting the time planners spend in the more adversarial and heavily scrutinised aspects of the occupation.

Such changes might, at least, allow for some change in the occupational culture of the profession, though of course they might not be desirable changes for other reasons.

PART V

Values in research

Introduction

Most professions these days see themselves as evidence-based and research aware. They require their members to base their practice on good evidence derived from research as well as to engage in well-informed reflective practice. They may also sponsor or encourage research that will help to inform professional activity.

In this section of the book, the nature of the values underlying and surrounding different kinds of research related to professional practice is explored. A more complex and tension-ridden picture than might at first be expected is revealed. The subject of values and research may appear narrow and specialised – a kind of metaphysical lacuna of concern and discourse which will only be of interest to those with an 'academic' bent. However, it will be seen that here, as elsewhere in this book, much can be learned generally about the relations of values and practice by taking a sideways look from what initially may seem a very particular perspective.

This volume has mostly been compiled by researchers in a variety of different disciplines. It is only right that there should be a part of the book where we self-consciously and critically reflect upon the relation of values to our own professional practice. What are the values that we as individuals and members of occupational groups espouse and embody in research work? And how are these values affected and modified by matters of context, client need and personal interest? The consideration of these questions is far from academic in that it has implications for us all as sponsors, producers and users of research. The following two chapters adopt different but complementary approaches to thinking about the place of values in research related to professional practice.

In Chapter 12 'Values and research: the case of nursing', Paul Wainwright and Ben Hannigan, two nurse educators with empirical and philosophical disciplinary backgrounds, respectively, reflect on the kind of research than can best serve a particular professional practice. The authors suggest that agreeing upon the kind of research that will best enable nursing practice to flourish and discharge its responsibilities is difficult. The nursing task is a complex, pluriform one. It involves the use of both natural scientific and more humanistic qualitative knowledge and data and insights.

Wainwright and Hannigan highlight the different, sometimes contradictory, values that underlie research in 'objective' scientific disciplines that theoretically underpin some nursing practices, and those that will help nurses to appreciate the subjective and 'soft' aspects of patient care. Nurses must serve the values of helping to combat disease through scientifically efficacious methods and ministering to the personal needs of the ill person via the use of good humanistic processes. In this context, they need to manage conflicting values and methods to attain beneficent outcomes for ill people.

This is not an easy task in practice; it raises complex questions about the relevance and types of research that should form the core of the disparate area designated 'nursing research'. Conceptual value issues implicit in research practice are thus shown to have substantial implications for a much larger debate about the nature of nursing practice and identity, a topic which is of immediate relevance to sufferers and carers on a daily basis. An academic discussion of the nature and implications of values underlying research thus transmutes into a much wider discussion about practical care in healthcare institutions and the role of individual health professionals. One of the most important implications here is that the values underlying academic methods and disciplines cannot usefully be discussed without constant reference to the needs and values of practitioners working under immediate pragmatic imperatives.

Roisin Pill has been an academically based professional empirical researcher, undertaking a variety of different kinds of healthcare-related research, for most of her working life. From this academic research location, in Chapter 13 'Professional researchers: values in the work context' she reflects personally upon some of the general and particular value issues that arise for researchers individually and as a group in conducting social research.

Building on a guiding assumption that no research can be value-free so the whole of the research process is shot through with value issues and commitments, Pill outlines the sorts of professional values that all researchers ideally might be deemed to share if their work is to flourish. These are honesty, courage, justice, objectivity, open-mindedness, collaboration and collegiality. Pill then goes on to show how these personal and professional values, together with the professionalised work culture they support, come under pressure from various quarters.

In particular, she shows how imminent and less immediate factors within and around the academic context of contemporary managed higher education can lead to radical changes in professional identity, values and choices in the name of expedient pragmatism. In this context, some important aspects of professional values and culture are under threat. Unfortunately, the researchers themselves are not necessarily in a good position to analyse and understand their predicament, nor to respond proactively to avoid some of the negative consequences of changes that might be thrust upon them without their active thought or consent. Pill concludes that researchers themselves need to do far more work on their own values and culture, and also to engage with other professional groups in comparative work.

A number of general issues arise from these two reflections on the relations between research and values. In the first place, it is clear that research as an activity in itself is shot through with values and value-related issues. Research projects, methods and their eventual findings are permeated with values of different kinds, whether researchers are conscious of this or not. Perhaps then it might be important to examine much more carefully which values should be selected and served by researchers, both in terms of ultimate aims and in relation to the appropriateness of particular methods in relation to specific projects and professional needs. As both chapters show, it is unlikely that research and researchers can be, or would aspire to be, value-free. That is not to say, however, that researchers have no choice in the values they adopt in their fundamental orientation and particular projects.

Just as particular research orientations and methods cannot be value-free, neither can they be insulated from external value pressures and influences emerging from social and professional needs, both intrinsic and extrinsic. Values and the practices they support come under intense pressure from various kinds of contextual and interest group pressures and imperatives. Researchers do not exist within a bubble of pure values that are independent of social context. There is, therefore, a complex dialogue, perhaps mostly tacit, between the values of the various stakeholders whose interests impinge upon research and researchers. This dialogue perhaps needs to become overt and more critical rather than remaining implicit or *sotto voce*.

Raising the question of the values that researchers serve and promulgate also raises important issues about the personal and corporate identity and nature of researchers as individuals and as a group. If researchers are not value-free collectors of evidence with an Olympian detachment from the messy world of values in professional practice, then how should they regard and orient themselves professionally? What sort of professionals should they be and what should their values be? Like any other professionals, they need to engage directly with the value content and aspirations of their own lives and activity. In this sense, they need to get their hands dirty. Or rather, they need to realise that their hands are already dirty – and far dirtier than they might like to hope. All of which suggests that researchers might research and understand the values informing their own practice more self-consciously and thoroughly without disappearing into a self-reflexive vortex.

The discussion of values in applied professional research initiated in the two chapters here thus leads to discussion of the values in professional practice and then to issues of professional identity and purpose for those who commission, undertake and use the findings of research. This is not a surprising conclusion in the context of this book. It is, however, an important one. Its implications need to be explored at far greater depth by members of the research 'guild' in critical discussion with each other and with those whose lives and work are potentially affected by their work.

CHAPTER 12

Values in research: the case of nursing

Paul Wainwright and Ben Hannigan

Introduction

In the 12-month period ending in March 2002, the UK's Nursing and Midwifery Council (NMC) reported that over 644 000 individuals had their names on the UK register of nurses, midwives and health visitors (NMC 2002b). Nurses therefore represent slightly more than 1% of the total UK population (Cowley 1999). In all areas of the UK, National Health Service (NHS) nurses form the largest part of the healthcare workforce. In terms of its cost to the UK economy, nursing consumes 3% of gross domestic product (Black 2002). Given this, 'it is astonishing how little investment has been and continues to be made in research on nursing, midwifery and health visiting' (Black 2002: ix).

Evidence submitted to the Higher Education Funding Council for England (HEFCE) and to the Department of Health suggests that only 3.9% of nursing academics are categorised as research staff; in addition, it has been estimated that there are 1600 nurses for every researcher whose salary costs are supported by funding obtained from a UK research council (HEFCE 2001). In repeated UK research selectivity exercises, in which the peer review of the outputs of academic departments has been used to determine future research funding, nursing research has fared badly in comparison with other, more established, disciplines. Just four UK university departments of nursing achieved ratings of 5 in the 2001 Research Assessment Exercise (RAE), whilst none achieved the top rating of 5*.

However, this rather dismal sketch of the state of nursing research tells only part of the story. From a relatively low base, research productivity within the discipline of nursing is continuing to grow. It is now widely accepted within nursing that research findings, alongside the accumulated personal knowledge developed through reflective practice, represent one of the most important forms of knowledge on which nursing care ought to be based. Whilst relatively few nurses may be producers of research, all nurses are now expected to be research consumers.

There are, however, substantial disagreements about the type of research required to underpin nursing practice and its place within the tradition of health services research. In this chapter, we consider the relationships between values and beliefs about knowledge, the nature of health, disease and illness, and research in nursing. We also address the ways in which research and research values impact on the identity of nursing and nurses.

Recent developments in nursing practice and education

We see nursing as an interpersonal activity, the central purpose of which is to promote the health, well-being and flourishing of individuals, families and communities. The main focus for medicine is the diagnosis of disease and the prescription of appropriate treatment to cure or palliate the condition. Nursing, on the other hand, claims to work at the level of the person and the person's response to the experience of illness. Nurses are united in pursuing this aim, although the practice settings in which they work will vary. In addition, many practitioners see this central purpose as representing an implicit contract between them and wider society (Avis 1999). Many nurses have worked hard to assert the independence of their practice from medicine, striving to develop models and theories that capture the distinct characteristics of the nursing contribution to healthcare (see McKenna 1997).

An important development in the UK in the 1970s and 1980s was the emergence of the 'new nursing' (Salvage 1990). This represented a sustained reaction against task-oriented, medically dominated and fragmented modes of care provision. The 'new nursing' promised a radical redefinition of the role of nurses, and of relationships between nurses and patients, and between nurses and doctors (Allen 2001). At its heart lay a belief in the significance of the therapeutic interpersonal relationship. Many nurses were no longer satisfied with roles that were limited to the administration of medically prescribed care, and instead came to see their work as explicitly encompassing a concern for the whole person.

These new ways of thinking about, and undertaking, nursing have been significant in a number of ways. First, the emphasis on holism and the pursuit of nursing as a therapeutic activity helped to underline the importance of the *process* of nursing care. The 'new nursing' explicitly encouraged practitioners to develop ways of working which transcended the delivery of technical interventions. The 'new nursing' and its attendant ideologies and practices also played a significant part in the progress towards professionalisation (Allen 2001). New ways of practising nursing demanded a new approach to the preparation of nurses, and the generation of a new and expanded knowledge base – including a knowledge base informed by increased research activity.

The Project 2000 curriculum, launched at the end of the 1980s, represented the fruition of this drive for a new approach to the education and training of nurses (United Kingdom Central Council for Nursing, Midwifery and Health Visiting [UKCC] 1986). Along with the introduction of Project 2000, NHS reforms introduced by the government of the day resulted in nursing education, in its entirety, moving into the higher education sector. Ideological commitment to the separation of purchaser and provider meant that district health authorities could no longer manage schools of nursing. The traditional apprenticeship-style preparation, in which students largely learned to nurse on the job, was supplanted by a university-based education in which qualifying nurses received both professional and academic accreditation. It is significant to note that, whilst the Project 2000 initiative has recently been replaced by a system of pre-qualifying education and training that more explicitly embraces the acquisition of nursing 'competencies' (UKCC 1999), this latest review of nursing preparation has not called into question the need for nursing education to be located in the higher education sector.

Research and nursing

On the basis of this preamble, we now turn our attention to a more specific analysis of the character and social organisation of nursing knowledge and nursing research. We consider, in particular, how the value ascribed to different forms of knowledge, including different forms of research knowledge, has come to exert a powerful influence on the character of the discipline of nursing and on nursing practice.

One of the difficulties we face is that research of interest or relevance to nurses and nursing falls into several different categories. Indeed, it is debatable whether there is any such thing as specifically 'nursing research'. For example, in the context of the 'new nursing' and the emphasis on the therapeutic content of nursing, there might be research into the nature of the interpersonal process that characterises nursing. This would require studies that address the necessary conditions for human well-being and flourishing so that we might identify the types of interventions we would require if we were to promote such flourishing. However, whether this should be characterised as 'nursing research', or whether it would more properly be called, for example, 'health philosophy', is a moot point.

Similarly, research into wound care, a key nursing responsibility, might involve laboratory studies of tissue viability, or the effect of maggots in tissue debridement, but such work would probably sit within a department of human physiology or bioscience. There is a similar problem for research into the type of interpersonal interventions that help people with severe mental health problems such as schizophrenia. This is an area of considerable importance to nurses working in the mental health field, but investigations of this sort may, more properly, fall under the umbrella of 'psychological research'. Nurses work with drugs, but the necessary knowledge comes under the science of pharmacology, while the prevention of decubitus ulcers, or joint contractures, in the immobile patient might come under biomechanics.

However, given our earlier comments about the desire of many nurses to professionalise their occupation (through, for example, developing theories of nursing, and through laying claim to a distinct and independent sphere of 'nursing' practice), and the move into higher education, it is not surprising that many academic nurses would wish to claim that there is such a thing as 'nursing' research. After all, if there are to be university departments of nursing, and if there is to be a nursing panel in the research assessment exercise (RAE), and if funding is to be identified to pay for research in nursing departments to be submitted to the RAE, then there must be pressure to have a body of work that can be called 'nursing research'. However, nursing appears to lack many of the characteristics of an academic research discipline.

Admittedly, the very idea of an academic discipline is a social construction. Knowledge does not come ready-sorted into convenient categories. It is placed (for the convenience of scholars and usually by scholars) into categories invented for the purpose. If there was a consensus that a new discipline of nursing should be created, it would, other things being equal, be possible. But a consideration of the nature of academic disciplines would suggest that if we did invent such a new discipline, it might be thought to have little in common with others.

The 'discipline' of nursing and the generation of knowledge for nursing practice

The shaping of knowledge into disciplines stems, as do so many things, from the ideas of Aristotle. He suggested a hierarchy of subjects, under the headings of theoretical (theology, mathematics and physics), practical (ethics and politics) and productive (the fine arts, poetics and engineering) (Moran 2002). Philosophy was held to be the universal field of enquiry that brought the rest together. According to Moran:

> The development and consolidation of the disciplines in the modern era was fundamentally related to both the growth of the universities and the increasing complexity of European societies.
> (Moran 2002: 4)

The need to relate education to economic and political ends resulted in the term 'discipline' being applied to professions such as medicine, law and theology. However, at least up to the end of the eighteenth century, under-graduates began their studies by following a liberal education before going on to specialise in their chosen profession. (Medical education in the USA and Canada is today entirely a postgraduate matter. There is an increasing trend in this direction in the UK.)

The inferior subjects in Aristotle's hierarchy, the productive disciplines of the fine arts, poetics and engineering, differ from the other two categories. Their objectives have less to do with the pursuit of knowledge than with the manufacture of artefacts. Today engineering would seem to typify the idea of an applied subject. Engineers apply the laws of mathematics, physics and material sciences to produce functional structures. Similarly, medicine, described in Moran's analysis as a profession rather than an academic subject, involves the application of the theoretical sciences of anatomy, physiology, biochemistry, microbiology, pharmacology and so on to the diagnosis and treatment by doctors of their patients' problems. The genera-tion of the knowledge used in these professions comes from research done in the theoretical disciplines.

Nursing is clearly not an academic, theoretical discipline like maths or physics. Its purpose is not the development of knowledge but the relief of suffering and the promotion of well-being. However, it does have much in common with the productive subjects because it involves the professional application of knowledge, borrowed from the theoretical subjects, to the production of solutions to the problems of patients. Like medicine, nursing makes use of knowledge from the natural sciences; for many nurses scien-tific research is highly valued.

However, if the objective of nursing is essentially about maximising the potential of patients, fostering well-being, providing nurture and so on, nurses need types of knowledge and ways of knowing other than those generated using only natural science research methods. If we accept the distinction between disease and illness, and accept for example that it is perfectly possible for a patient to be diagnosed as having a clinical pathology and yet to feel quite well and, conversely, to have their pathology corrected and yet still to feel unwell (Greaves 1996, and see also below for more detailed discussion), we need a richer understanding than that which can be provided by the natural sciences, and by the biomedical sciences in parti-cular.

The difficulty stems, at least in part, from the philosophical basis for the natural sciences and, particularly, for biomedicine. The rationale for the randomised controlled trial, which is widely recognised in hierarchies of evidence in the evidence-based medicine arena as the gold standard for knowledge, is specifically designed so as to eliminate the human element from the investigation. Since the rise of empiricism in the seventeenth century the natural sciences have permitted themselves the study only of that which can be empirically observed, supposedly to the exclusion of human preferences, intentions, purposes and values. The assumption in clinical trials is that it is the lesion that can be treated, regardless of the state of mind of the sufferer. Trials are based on the premise that an identical treatment is given to a sample of patients, while a competing treatment or an inactive placebo is given to a population statistically similar in all important respects, with neither subjects nor researchers knowing which group is which. Objective measures are taken of the relevant outcomes and any improvement demonstrated in the performance of the new agent is assumed to be generalisable to all other sufferers.

The shortcomings of this approach are evident even within the relatively narrow realms of research into disease and pathology. To place such methods at the head of a hierarchy of evidence, as if quantitative research should be acknowledged as quite simply 'better' than any other way of knowing about anything, seems little short of folly. Writers such as Oakley (2000), Pickstone (2000) and Midgely (2001) have all argued that we need a far richer and more complex account of ways of knowing than can be offered by the natural sciences alone.

Debates about 'ways of knowing' resonate in nursing. Some nurses have maintained that natural science research methods, akin to those which dominate medical research, should be the clear methods of choice in generating knowledge for nursing practice. Gournay (1999) proposes seven reasons in support of this position, including putting forward a case for the randomised controlled trial as the best way to produce evidence of the 'effectiveness' of nursing work. Important nursing studies of this type exist, and are – reflecting the dominance of the idea of 'hierarchies of evidence' – often held up as the 'best' examples of nursing research (*see*, for example, Gournay and Brooking 1994).

However, many nurses have adopted what might generally be called qualitative methods to investigate human experience. If the challenge for nurses is to understand the patient's experience of illness, what would seem to be required would be an account that was ideographic, i.e. acknowledging the unique character of particular events, rather than nomothetic, i.e. seeking the identification of universal laws (Hammersley 1989). Thus many nurses have adopted approaches to research that draw on the traditions of ethnography, or hermeneutics, or phenomenology, or similar methodologies. For example, Barker *et al.* (1999) have used qualitative methodologies as a means of generating knowledge relating to the 'need for psychiatric nursing'. Some nurses have even made the case that a degree of natural 'fit' exists between the focus of nursing and the focus of qualitative research (*see*, for example, Cutcliffe and Goward 2000).

Paradigms for health, illness and research

Disputes in nursing over the 'right' way to generate knowledge for practice are also related to differing perspectives for understanding the nature of 'health', 'disease' and 'illness'. The key point to grasp here is that, at the level of both the individual and society, various sets of beliefs (and their associated behaviours) can and do exist simultaneously. We may accept this is true for other cultures but be less ready to accept the implications for our own society because of the predominance of Western biomedicine. Yet a moment's reflection will reveal that, in addition to traditional folk and lay prescriptions for maintaining health and treating disease, there are a wide range of alternative medical paradigms in Britain today; practitioners of alternative therapies flourish in every town. Thus the particular set of health beliefs held by an individual at a single point in time could be coloured by age, ethnicity, level of education, family attitudes, and their experience of varied biomedical and alternative practitioners. This is as true for health professionals as for the general public.

It should not, therefore, be surprising that there are differing views among nurses that affect their ideas about how to generate knowledge for practice. Moreover, even within the current system of beliefs associated with Western biomedicine, there is room for practitioners to exercise choice in the way they practise and the approach they might adopt to research, depending on the particular emphasis they place on maintaining health or treating disease.

Ideas from ancient Greece about health, illness and disease shaped medieval practice and laid the foundations for contemporary secular medicine. It has been argued that the dominant paradigm of reductionist biomedicine, with its emphasis on disease, is constantly challenged by other paradigms, for example the perspectives of social medicine and public health. Several writers have commented that the ancient Greek medical tradition revealed this tension between a collectivist and an individualistic approach (Dubos 1960; Greaves 1996; Turner 2000).

This was symbolised in the mythology surrounding the two figures of Hygeia, associated with the virtues of a rational life in a pleasant and healthy environment, and Asclepius, the first physician who promotes an interventionist medicine that restores health by directly treating the ailments of an individual. Dubos claims that, in one form or another, these complementary emphases in medicine have always existed simultaneously in all civilisations.

Biomedicine defines health and illness largely in terms of biologically based diseases. It is a perspective that treats the ill person, often by default, as a biological object; here, health is defined in terms of absence of disease (Armstrong 2000: 27ff). This is contrasted with perspectives that emphasise a holistic view of the individual where health is defined in terms of a person's ability to realise their vital goals. The focus is on the individual as a social being and their *experience of disease*, i.e. their illness.

In their ideas as to what constitutes both good nursing practice and good nursing research, different nurses have placed varying degrees of emphasis on whether the focus of nursing should be on the 'disease' or the 'illness'. We consider it no coincidence that nurses more closely associated with natural science methodologies tend to place greater store on the importance of the former.

Gournay (2003), for example, argues for a form of nursing which directly attends to the underlying disease that 'inhabits' the sick person; in this formulation, administering medication may be the most important activity that nurses can undertake. Barker and colleagues (1997), on the other hand, make the argument that disease *per se* has never been of central interest to nurses. Rather, 'nursing's task is, and has always been, to help people deal with the human problems they experience' (Barker *et al.* 1997: 660). In this formulation, nursing practice and research should pay less heed to 'disease' and more to the individual's response to this.

It is tempting to suggest that nursing fits much more comfortably into the Hygeian model of health and illness, as a counterbalance to the Asclepian view of the world favoured by medicine. However, this would be to fall into an obvious trap. For one thing, as we have already suggested, many nurses want to draw from biomedicine in their treatment of clinical conditions. From a pragmatic point of view, medical science can give us effective tools to relieve specific symptoms or to treat infections. We would be foolish to deny ourselves and our patients their use. At the very least, we would be advised to operate a judicious mix of the two approaches.

However, this approach still has its problems. Neither account is sufficient to cope with the problems of modern healthcare. Simply adding them together will not solve the problem. The patient's experience as the sufferer, and the doctor's or nurse's experience as the clinician, will be informed and shaped by their respective experiences and value systems. These experiences will be constantly changing and being reformulated. This means that illness becomes less a matter of taxonomy and more, as Good (1994) suggests, a matter of the interpretation of a narrative, akin to the reading of a novel or a play. All the readers or watchers will construct the story and create the characters for themselves and each account will be different.

Values, research and nursing

It is clear throughout the foregoing account that values are critical to our understanding of nursing practice and the research related to it. Nursing, it seems, needs to utilise appropriate technical knowledge. At the same time, it must acknowledge the importance of human experience and the human response to illness.

It is sometimes argued that the natural sciences are somehow 'value-free', that they provide a standard of objectivity necessarily absent from qualitative research. In our view this is a myth. The decision to study only those natural objects that can be observed empirically and to attempt to exclude all aspects of human preferences or intentions is itself an expression of a value; this value judgement is restated every time a randomised controlled trial is designed and conducted.

So powerful is this value system that, as Midgely (2001) suggests, it has led many to claim that scientific methods are the only rational way to understand any topic, including social and psychological enquiries. This attitude has provoked what is sometimes called an anti-science feeling, not uncommon among some nurses, a feeling that Midgely suggests is:

> a protest against [scientific] imperialism – a revulsion against the way of thinking which deliberately extends the impersonal, reductive, atomistic methods that are appropriate to physical sciences into social and psychological enquiries where they work badly.
>
> (Midgely 2001:1)

But to what extent is nursing, or the knowledge required for effective nursing, scientific? Again, as Midgely points out, it depends what you mean by 'scientific'. On the one hand the word can mean no more than thorough, or methodical (and we would probably want nursing to adopt that as a value system). On the other hand, it can mean in a strictly factual sense 'concerned with the natural sciences' (Midgely 2001: 144). From the latter perspective, the important aspects of nursing that have to do with interpersonal relationships and the understanding of the personal response to illness and suffering clearly have nothing to do with natural science and are explicitly ruled out of consideration by the natural sciences. This area of practice requires a very different kind of knowledge and different ways of knowing. As many nurses have argued, nurses require self-knowledge to function effectively and with compassion in their interpersonal relationships with patients.

Midgely has also suggested that we find it difficult to understand our own behaviour and that of other people. However, even in everyday life we have to make the attempt. As she says:

> Total ignorance about our own motives, habits and capacities is not excusable. Knowledge about these things is not an optional subject ... which we can drop if we are not very good at it. Failure to know ourselves can be a serious moral fault. And one reason why it is a fault is that it blocks our understanding of other people.
>
> (Midgely 2001: 145)

We would argue that nursing requires an understanding of others and that this, in turn, requires the nurse to show empathy and sympathy. To do this, it is necessary that nurses are attentive to their own motives and reactions. Such attention is not just a matter of good technique, but rather a profoundly moral requirement; as Carper (1978) suggests, the nurse is required to be a certain kind of person. Thus the pursuit of knowledge for nursing practice, far from being a value-free, scientific quest for objectivity, is actually inextricably bound up in a complex system of values and subjective enquiry.

This imperative appears to be accepted by many nurses. Many, for example, have embraced the notion of the 'reflective practitioner', and the associated idea that the accumulated personal wisdom of the experienced clinician is an invaluable source of knowledge for nursing practice.

Conclusion

At the very least, nursing has a difficult balancing act to perform. Nurses need to make use of science and scientific facts. To pretend that they do not sounds rather odd. After all, we cannot put the kettle on to make a comforting cup of tea for a patient without making use of natural science. But if we believe that an understanding of human experience and a desire to promote human flourishing are necessary components of nursing, then science alone will not do. Somehow, nurses have to find a way to integrate their understanding of science with their humanitarian function as carers. In doing this, they must exhibit the human virtues and knowledge appropriate to this role.

With regard to the future for 'nursing research', we note that the future of all university-based research activity in the UK is currently under review, underpinned by a clear message from central government that a more selective approach to funding will be introduced. Less mature research disciplines, like nursing, may find that an already harsh research-funding environment becomes harsher still. Given the concern with clinical effectiveness and evidence-based practice, this environment is likely to be more sympathetic to research into technologies, taking a natural science approach, than to qualitative studies that seek to understand therapeutic human interaction.

Differing perspectives within nursing with respect to the nature of health, disease and illness and with the focus of nursing practice will continue to shape the characteristics of nursing research and the nature of nursing knowledge. We suspect that nurses will continue to produce research that reflects a variety of paradigms, and that individual practitioners will draw on this in a manner that reflects their own values and interests. The wider challenge remains: how can nursing, and the other healthcare professions, integrate the quantitative and qualitative paradigms? Healthcare in general needs an epistemology that can bring together the apparently irreconcilable perspectives of Hygeia and Asclepius. It may be that this can come only from an interdisciplinary approach in which disputes about 'nursing research' or 'medical research' are subsumed under a broader research programme.

CHAPTER 13

Professional researchers: values in the work context

Roisin Pill

Introduction

Research (defined as literary or scientific enquiry) is an activity that has traditionally been associated with the universities, the gatekeeper institutions to professional status. While many researchers can be found working for private organisations and companies, the vast majority in the UK still work for public higher education institutions. It will be argued here that research is a professional activity and an important aspect of professional practice. It is, therefore, a place where one might *expect* to see professional values being made overt and enacted.

There has been considerable debate about the nature of the relationship between values and research. Few scientists would now argue that research can be 'value-free' and totally objective. Most would recognise that values enter into the research process, if only in the selection of the topic. Researcher values influence the identification of certain problems and the ways in which they are then studied. The commitment to attaining scientific objectivity (or rigorous method) is itself a value commitment.

However, researchers do differ in their views about the role that values play in the research process (May 2001: 46ff). Some claim that it is possible to be 'objective' in the collection and analysis of data. Their critics maintain that social research is not a neutral medium for generating information on social realities; it constructs rather than unveiling 'facts'. Since the researcher plays a major role in this activity, a fuller discussion of what is good – that is, what values guide researchers in their studies and interventions – is required.

> Simply 'knowing about' the issues of values and ethics is not a sufficient basis upon which to conduct research; they need to

form part of research practice itself. ... Many now argue that an examination of the basis of values and their relationship to decisions and stages in research is required in order to provide justification for systematic and valid social research. The aim is not their elimination, for this is impossible. Instead, these criticisms acknowledge that research takes place within a context where certain interests and values often predominate to the exclusion of others. 'Objective' research is not then achieved by uncritically accepting these as self-evident.

(May 2001: 67)

In the material which follows, I will adopt the fundamental assumption that the practice of research is shot through with values, value choices and value commitments at all points. Thus the types of research that are selected, the methods that are used and the ends to which research is eventually put are value-laden.

A view from the inside

After several false starts in trying to write about the topic of researchers' values and the various pressures and conflicts that could influence and distort them, it gradually became clear to me that the best way to proceed was to reflect on my own experiences and observations of others in a similar position. Although I have spent all my working life to date as a researcher with a background in the social sciences (medical sociology and anthropology), I found this surprisingly difficult to do and a salutary experience. (This, incidentally, confirms one of our original findings, that professionals do not often think about their values and are inclined to take them for granted!)

The following pages present the reflections upon values of someone who has spent her life almost entirely in university departments (apart from a one-year fling with a well-known market research company) and has carried out research almost exclusively in the field of health and illness. It is a personal view of the values that I think underpin the researcher role, those that I consider most important and 'most valuable' personally. Nevertheless, being a social scientist by training, it was inevitable that I should also start to analyse and bring sociological concepts to bear on the account I was producing.

This chapter, therefore, attempts to cover two linked themes: first, some personal reflections on the values held by social researchers and the contextual factors that erode or facilitate their expression; secondly, some sociological speculation on the importance of the culture of the work setting for professional values.

Reflections on values and the social researcher

What, then, do I value most in my professional role? My preliminary answers are these:

- the freedom to decide how to carry out the work and organise my time
- doing work that is intellectually demanding and of interest to other colleagues in my discipline
- doing work that has a practical and worthwhile purpose for others
- the satisfaction of carrying a study through to a successful conclusion and having the work recognised by peers and those funding it.

Like many other professionals, it is autonomy in the workplace and the quality of relationships with peers and clients that I most value.

Autonomy is one of the many traits that is nearly always put forward in both popular and specialist discourse about professions. Professional workers have been taught to expect to make independent 'professional' judgements about proper courses of action in their sphere of expertise. Researchers, whatever their disciplinary background, expect and value the freedom to discuss ideas and share data with their peer networks, to use their expert knowledge to design a study using methods that they deem to be most appropriate, and to publish and disseminate their findings without any constraint. Throughout history, freedom of thought and expression have been valued and denied in equal measure. They are particularly important values to those purporting to be dedicated to knowledge and the pursuit of truth and are generally espoused by academics of every discipline.

When thinking about the underlying values, explicit and implicit, that would be accepted unquestioningly by all professional researchers and expected by the rest of society, one inevitably comes back to the trinity of *honesty, courage* and *justice (equity)*. These are the fundamental principles that provide the basis for the moral probity of any profession (Friedson 1970) and the possibility of practitioners acting in virtuous ways. I will spell out what this might mean in practice specifically for researchers in their relationships with peers and clients.

Honesty

All professional researchers owe a duty to their employers to carry out the study in a competent manner, to report the findings accurately and to show appropriate caution and balance in drawing any conclusions. However, technical competence is not enough. They must also be people of integrity in whom trust can be reposed by the relevant stakeholders, e.g. employers, funding bodies, the wider academic community and anyone else who may be affected by their work. This means they must be honest.

The most heinous crime that a researcher could commit would be to fabricate or falsify results. Equally reprehensible would be the deliberate omission of relevant evidence in any argument being put forward, or the alteration of the findings for extrinsic purposes. However, this is where another value becomes important, namely, readiness to be open-minded and consider other possibilities – a capacity to remain aware that there are always other ways of seeking answers to questions and pursuing knowledge which may be equally valid. For the researcher, this is closely linked to honesty and integrity. *Honesty* and *openness of mind* are key implicit and normative values that are likely to be expected by the wider society and to be celebrated in the rhetoric about researchers.

Courage

Under what circumstances might a researcher be expected to demonstrate courage? This value is linked very closely to honesty. One needs courage, for example, to resist temptations to cut corners, to fabricate data or to slant the reporting of findings to suit a sponsor's preconceptions. Such internal pressure may be resisted by feelings of pride in one's work and self-esteem, i.e. by a strong personal value being placed on the quality of one's work and one's professional identity. Pressure to be less than scrupulous may also be external, emanating from colleagues, superiors or funding bodies. It is likely to vary in the level of explicitness. Furthermore, it is *perceived* pressure, whether or not it actually exists, that affects action.

Courage is also needed in cases of inappropriate, unprofessional and illegal behaviour observed in others. It may be necessary for researchers to become 'whistle-blowers' if they witness certain kinds of practices and behaviours among their colleagues. These include scientific fraud on the part of colleagues, work where there is the possibility of physical or psychological harm being done to research subjects/respondents, and situations where there has been inappropriate recruitment of people to a study or inadequate measures have been put in place to ensure that full informed consent has been obtained.

Justice

Courage may also be needed by the researchers who place high value on ensuring that justice (equity) is manifested in their work and relationships with research subjects and colleagues. They may feel obliged to ask awkward questions about the way junior staff or potentially vulnerable respondents are being treated in the course of a research project.

Commitment to the value of justice also arises in the unequal relationship that may exist between researchers and their subjects. Researchers have attempted to deal with this in two main ways. There has been a strong tradition, particularly among sociologists and feminist scholars, in which researchers have seen themselves as being on the side of the underdog, giving a voice to the dispossessed, deviant, disabled, disadvantaged and powerless (Becker 1970b; Oakley 1980). Some researchers have thus seen their role as one of advocate, or, at least, making sure that the views of their research subjects are put forward as accurately and fairly as possible so others, often health or social care professionals, can appreciate the real concerns, perceptions and problems of their clients.

A more radical development of this position has been to move towards regarding research as a collaborative, appreciative process in which potential respondents are invited to take part directly in identifying the questions and methods that should be included in any project (Reason 1994). This allows for a de-objectification of research subjects and much greater equality between researchers and members of the public. However, the practicalities of involving people directly in the research process in this way are considerable. Reason notes:

> As soon as we touch upon the question of participation we have to entertain and *work with* issues of power, of oppression, of gender; we are confronted with the limitations of our skill, with the rigidities of our own and others' behaviour patterns, with the other pressing demands on our limited time, with the hostility or indifference of our organisational contexts. We live out our contradictions, struggling to bridge the gap between our dreams and reality, to realise the values we espouse.
>
> (Reason 1994: 2)

Factors that contribute to the erosion of researcher values

Reason's comment brings us back to reality with a bump. While researchers may personally aspire to, and even often enact, the fundamental virtues of honesty, courage and justice described above, their capacity to do this is affected by context. I will now consider the significant wider factors that bear upon the professional researcher's values.

Brint notes that there is a:

> constant juxtaposition of freedom and constraint on professional work: the simultaneous experience of a large degree of technical control over work and, often, a significant degree of opportunity combined with the constraints of organisational life and the fluctuations of market demand for expert labour.
>
> (Brint 1994: 12)

The key words here are 'organisation' and 'market'. The former draws attention to the micro-level of the immediate work setting and the latter to the macro-level of the larger political and economic forces that inevitably affect these organisations. Both the micro- and the macro-level need to be kept in mind when considering the ways in which professionals are able to put their values into practice.

The majority of professionals today work in organisations. In these settings they will assume tasks and responsibilities and be assigned a position depending on their level of expertise and experience. The typical organisational hierarchy with its systems of accountability and control may appear to conflict with the concept of the professional as a competent autonomous individual, who, once they have been selected and have the credentials to practice, can do so as an equal of others in the same profession – a colleague rather than a subordinate. Nevertheless, this is the challenge that faces the newly qualified professional. They must fit in to a particular work context and attempt to reconcile personal and professional values with the practices they observe. The culture of the employing organisation is therefore crucial. Here, focusing on social researchers, I shall attempt to suggest exactly which features of their work contexts make it more or less supportive to their implicit and expressed values and subsequent behaviour.

The immediate work context in higher education

In what ways might the culture of the employing organisation – the immediate work context – contradict, modify or support researcher values? In the case of many social researchers, the employing organisation is likely to be a higher education institution committed to traditional academic values, the fostering of scholarship and the pursuit of knowledge. The following remarks are based on experience of researchers in universities.

The ideal setting for research and a researcher to flourish is one where there are others with whom work can be discussed easily and openly, and where colleagues and junior staff can be supportive to each other, sharing expertise and giving constructive advice. A setting that actively encourages collegial interaction like this facilitates self-regulation and scrutiny of the work of others in a natural way, so honesty, courage and equity have more chance of proliferating. This enables researchers to establish relations of confidence and trust with their peers. Such 'professionalised work environments' are characterised by high levels of education and an orientation to formal knowledge among staff and management.

This kind of open, trusting, respectful, collegial, egalitarian culture is more conducive to high morale and self-esteem than one typified by prescriptive external bureaucratic checks and regulation. Free movement of ideas and comments on work projects are vital to a creative, happy research culture. Like many other good things of value, like health and happiness, such a setting tends to be taken for granted. It is likely to be lamented and consciously appreciated only when it is no longer there!

One of the main pressures on the professionalised work culture and the values that sustain it is the need to find adequate resources. For individual researchers at department or unit level, as with so many professionals, the scarce resources are time and money.

Social scientists in a full-time academic post, like other academics, have to balance the demands of teaching and research. A perceived lack of time minimises the chance for discussions or the insights gleaned in casual conversation that can spark ideas and build teamwork and trust. Meetings may be difficult to arrange and poorly attended. Time not spent in preparing and writing papers for submission may be regarded as wasted. Without trusting relationships, which require time to develop, ideas may be guarded and not shared for fear of poaching and development by another. Ultimately, the value of research may be threatened because inadequate thought is devoted to planning and analysis in the rush to meet extrinsic deadlines.

Even if the resource of adequate time for developing relationships and ideas is available, most researchers are aware of the imperative to seek funding in order to get research going. Once a research project requires more than a single individual with access to a library, obtaining funding becomes an issue. Decisions have to be made about the *nature* of the research and *likely sources of support*. Each researcher must strike a balance between what they would like to work on and the topics currently or likely to be funded. Compromises will inevitably be made. Since most research contracts are short term (commonly two or three years), full-time researchers can find themselves on a treadmill of writing and submitting protocols that are acceptable to the overall plans of their current employing organisation as well as carrying out their current project.

Within social scientific research related to the health and policy spheres, for example, there may well be a conflict between the desire to undertake 'pure' research – a contribution to the theory and knowledge of an academic discipline which is basically the pursuit of knowledge and truth for its own sake – and 'applied' research – a contribution to understanding or solving a problem perceived by policy makers or practitioners. The tension between these two very different roles of social science research in the health field has been characterised as the difference between 'sociology *of* medicine' and 'sociology *in* medicine'. The former has been described as a 'tradition of social science, based on autonomous analytic academic disciplines, whose primary contribution is to provide social, cultural and political critiques on the nature of health and healthcare'. The latter is in a 'tradition of applied research typically attempting to provide useful evidence within the healthcare system while accepting the current institutional and other frameworks' (Albrecht *et al.* 2000: 3).

Increasingly, projects involve the use of mixed teams of researchers of varying levels of skill and ability together with other support workers. This, in turn, raises issues of quality control and the bureaucratisation of the research process. Researchers who are grant holders have to take on the responsibility of line-manager to support staff and often a supervisor role in relation to junior research staff. The responsibility they feel for the latter can also create pressures since there is concern about the end of the contract and whether it will be possible to keep people who have proved themselves on the payroll. The need to write a successful proposal within a relatively short time-span (and the compromises this may entail) can exert strong limitations on research design and creativity. There are pressures, therefore, to lean towards the safe option of a project designed to answer a current problem defined by a commissioning body, using methods that will be acceptable to them. Within this context, there may also be pressures to regard junior researchers as expendable 'hired hands' rather than colleagues.

Such pressures of lack of time and the constant need to look for funding and 'to be aware of the bottom line' are typical of many work settings in which professionals work. However, in the context of research work, the significance of resource-related pressures is that they tend to erode the possibility of maintaining a workplace culture that fosters a variety of research approaches and encourages trusting, co-operative rather than competitive, relations between researchers.

These corrosive trends are being exacerbated by the changing political, economic and social environment in which the employing organisations – the higher education institutions – find themselves.

Wider external factors contributing to erosion of researcher values in higher education

Beyond the immediate work context exerting its own pressures on research culture and values, there are a number of wider factors. These include the changing priorities and expectations of higher education institutions, the values of wider society in determining research funding priorities, the perceived need to make research applied and relevant, and the dominance of narrow 'scientific' paradigms for doing research.

Changing priorities and expectations in higher education

As part of the public sector, universities are under ever-increasing pressure to demonstrate value for money (Power 1997; *The Economist* 2003: 33). The higher education funding councils now make regular elaborate assessments of the quality of research. The subsequent level of funding allocated to universities and departments depends on the result of the research assessment ratings.

The Research Assessment Exercise (RAE) takes place every four years. It has had a marked effect on the pattern of research in the UK with some institutions no longer carrying out research in certain areas and departments being closed or amalgamated (Harley 2002; Hare 2003). Institutions have reacted to these pressures with a variety of strategies. Before the approaching RAE, researchers who have obtained large grants and have published widely in peer-reviewed journals are in demand. They may be 'head-hunted' by units keen to bolster their profile. Within departments, staff may be encouraged, or directed, to concentrate on particular research areas or themes selected by the institutional hierarchy as providing the best chance of producing highly rated publications and large amounts of external funding. For those heavily involved in research, these developments mean that personal preferences and expertise in a given topic may have to be ignored in favour of areas of work that are deemed best for the institution.

As noted earlier, substantial research projects increasingly involve a team of workers, often recruited specifically for that contract. The team has to be managed to achieve the goal of a successfully completed project within the resources and time-scale contracted. This, in turn, raises issues of quality control for the responsible researcher as grant holder. Competence, motivation and integrity cannot necessarily be assumed. Given the nature and constraints of the situation, the pressures to cut corners, fabricate or 'improve' data may be quite considerable both for junior and senior staff (Miller and Hersen 1992). Job security, future funding and career prospects within the employing organisation may all be perceived to be at stake.

It is not possible to quantify the extent of the threat that external pressures of this kind represent to traditional professional researcher culture with its values of honesty, courage and justice in social research. However, it is worth noting that in other areas of research where similar pressures exist, e.g. the biomedical field, research misconduct has been described as 'endemic' in the UK and the USA by the chairman of the Committee on Publication Ethics (COPE), a body of UK medical journal editors concerned with combating medical research fraud:

> Earlier this year the US office of Research Integrity, which deals only with research funded by the US Public Health Service, released a review of over 1000 allegations of scientific fraud, investigated between 1993 and 1997. The review, *Scientific Misconduct Investigations 1993–1997*, shows that falsification, fabrication and plagiarism were the most common findings.
>
> (The COPE Report 1999)

Wider social values

Apart from the immediate constraints being imposed by the institutions and the increasing bureaucratisation of the research process, the whole process of obtaining funding can further undermine researcher creativity and autonomy and reinforce the less constructive trends already described. The amount of money allocated and the type of research prioritised naturally reflects the values of the wider society. Thus it will come as no surprise that the allure of the biomedical sciences to public and private funding sources is enormous and that social science research in the health field has had very limited resources in comparison. This despite growing recognition of the need to complement biomedical with social scientific understanding of the nature of health and illness.

Within the field of health and healthcare, the impact of social values is clearly seen in the way that funding distribution reflects the perceived importance of certain categories of people. For example, traditionally, less has been spent on services and research for the patients of so-called Cinderella specialities, such as mental illness, learning disabilities and geriatrics, compared with other acute specialities. In the private sector, similar differences are to be observed in the reluctance of some of the big pharmaceutical companies to develop drugs for Third World diseases while concentrating on new variants of already existing drugs for the conditions most prevalent in Western industrial societies.

The bias towards 'applied' research

For social researchers the main source of funds is the government, either directly or through the research councils. Understandably, perhaps, there is a tendency to channel money towards more applied research work and to encourage social scientists to become part of a problem-solving system that seeks to explain, prevent, cure or manage disease or other social problems. The trend is to commission research on a particular topic. However, commissioning bodies rarely seek researchers' expert advice about questions that could usefully be investigated or the most appropriate methods. Their briefing documents tend to reflect their own values and assumptions in these matters, reducing professional autonomy and creativity. In response, researchers produce findings using a routine approach relying on a few well-tried methods and designs – a 'cookbook' approach to research. The temptation often is to use quantitative methods which can be carried out by a team and produce data that lends themselves to statistical analysis. (Other approaches, such as those employed in qualitative enquiry, rely much more on the individual skills of the researcher(s) who work together in a more collegiate and equal way.)

The implication is that social researchers concerned with maximising their chances for funding should consider writing proposals for topics decided by others and adopt standard methods to ensure greater simplicity in delivering the project. There are even greater incentives not to be too creative in their approach since then they increase the risk of falling at the first hurdle because of the way they conceptualise and propose to carry out the work. This brings us to the issue of research paradigms and the long shadow cast by the Western model of science, particularly the bio-sciences, over research of all kinds.

The dominance of narrow 'scientific' paradigms

In our society, 'scientific' explanations and 'facts' are commonly privileged as objective, universal public knowledge that explains the world around us and allows us to manipulate it better (Midgely 2001; Stivers 2001). The 'scientific method' informs common notions of what is considered as 'proper' research. It largely determines what are considered to be appropriate topics for investigation and the best ways to go about it as well as what counts as evidence and how to evaluate it. Such an emphasis on the virtues of the scientific method, narrowly understood, as opposed to other paradigms continues to have unfortunate consequences for researchers looking for funding. If reviewers and grant-giving committees are adherents of positivist science, they can be reluctant to fund proposals based on different epistemological and ontological assumptions.

Conclusion

In this chapter the starting assertion was that values are intertwined inextricably with every stage of the research process from inception of the study to dissemination of the findings. The aim was to use the topic of research to explore how the values of a particular professional group, the workplace, and the personal and professional values of the individual interact with each. The example used was that of social researchers in a university setting, using my own experience and observations as a guide. Having reflected on the values that I and my colleagues consider most important and the characteristics of the immediate work context that would be perceived as supportive of good research, I then suggested certain trends and external factors at societal level that could fundamentally change professional research culture and its basic espoused values of honesty, open-mindedness, courage, justice, equality, collaboration and collegiality.

In the context of their role as employees of institutions, academic researcher professionals, like many others, are now facing the pressures experienced in the real world where the market rules. In this context, the culture of the employing organisation is very important for social science researchers in influencing their values, choices and opportunities. Their professional organisations are weak, with no regulatory functions and limited membership, though they do issue guidance on a range of ethical matters concerning the conduct of research and duties to the subjects involved (Association of Social Anthropologists 2003; British Sociological Association 2003). Other researchers, such as those in the natural sciences and biomedical sciences, who have expert knowledge that is in short supply and sought by the private as well as the public sector will obviously be in a very different market situation and have correspondingly more opportunities.

What is missing from the above account are any firm data on how social researchers are currently coping with the pressures identified and the ways that they are actually affecting their values. The emphasis on powerful factors challenging professional culture and values might appear to suggest that professionals are somehow trapped and passively caught in a fixed role; they will *inevitably* succumb to the extrinsic pressures and the values of professional research culture will die.

This perspective is one-sided. It makes little provision for the possibility that individuals and groups may, by their choices, resist such trends and, by maintaining professional values, actively help to maintain and shape the context in which they work. Unfortunately, we presently have no detailed evidence of how structural changes affect the professional values held and enacted. Nor is there in the literature any adequate theorising about the role that professional ideologies play in the organisation and operation of professional fields (Nelson and Trubeck 1992: 15–27). Similarly, little attention has been paid to the world views that professionals develop in response to professional training, workplace pressures and the social and institutional context in which the workplace is embedded.

Social science researchers have often refuted common but ill-founded assumptions that there is a close correspondence between formal declarations of professional values, as in codes of professional ethics, and the values actually held by individuals, least of all in relation to their own professional group. But they have not gone on to explore, understand or explain the *nature* of the relationship. This suggests that there is a need for more studies of the workplace as a context that produces professional ideologies and values (Nelson and Trubeck 1992). We need a better, more pluralistic comparative framework that integrates studies of structural and organisational changes and factors with studies of the reactions and perceptions of those involved in such changing systems. This framework needs to pay far more attention to the implicit and explicit values of the professionals whose own personal and occupational values are caught up in the complex context and values of their employing organisations and the wider social context. Among the groups who should be studied more specifically are social researchers themselves.

Conclusion

CHAPTER 14

Professions and values: a dynamic relationship

Stephen Pattison and Roisin Pill

When we first started thinking about writing this book, our working title was *The Trouble with Values*. At that time, this best summed up the complex feelings aroused during our first attempts at producing drafts. They were a mixture of the following:

- exasperation at the 'slipperiness' of the subject
- frustration at the lack of previous work that had tried to relate values to professional practice in a variety of different contexts
- conviction about the importance of the topic
- desire to involve and engage others in this task.

The production of this book has not substantially altered these feelings – if anything, it has reinforced them.

Most readers will be familiar with the one-page mission and vision statements which often occupy prominent places in official organisational documents and communications (Talbot 2000). Perhaps this is one of the most familiar mechanisms whereby we are all reminded on a day-to-day basis that certain values are regarded as fundamental to working and professional life. The progenitors of mission statements often insist that they should be the locus of a continuing organisation-wide discussion which leads to constant revision: they are more likely to end up being ignored. Frequently, however, their fate is to be framed and solemnly hung up on entrance and office walls – or, even worse perhaps, to be laminated and pushed into a drawer or wallet and allowed to moulder quietly.

The life-cycle of the mission statement – from dynamic discussion to death by lamination – can perhaps be regarded as a parable of the position of discussion about values and professions today. On the face of it, it can seem that all professionals, professions and organisations want to do is to identify and adopt some rather general values then get on with business as usual, secure in the belief that they have done the 'right thing'.

If this book has established one thing, it is that a static, uncritical view of professions and values is simply not tenable in contemporary society and social institutions. The implication of this is that all of us – researchers, policy makers, members of organisations, professional legislators, educators and trainers, individual professionals and workers, or users of the services of professions and professionals – need to take more seriously the dynamic, conflicting and changing relationships which form the living ecology surrounding values and professions today.

In other words, *all* of us should become much more proactively conscious and curious about the nature and dynamics of values and professions. This will be intellectually interesting in its own right. But it is also necessary if we are to *choose and live out* some values rather than simply unconsciously and uncritically acting out the values of others in everyday life and practice.

In this final chapter, we will highlight some of the key themes and issues that arise from the contributions to this book as a whole. We will suggest some ways in which various groups and individuals might be able to engage further with these themes and issues. Then we go on to outline some ways in which further investigations into the dynamic relationships between professions and values might be pursued.

Key themes and issues

A main insight emerging from the various contributions to this book is that the relationship between professions and values is a vital, dynamic and continuously changing one. The concepts, professions and values, may often be taken at first sight to denote unchanging monolithic solidity. If values are invoked at all by professions and professionals, they are often talked of as if the same values have always been important to this particular group, have always occupied the same position, been interpreted in the same way, etc.

There are analogies with the experiences of anthropologists among more exotic tribes who, when enquiring of their respondents *why* they did things a certain way, were often somewhat frustrated to receive the answer 'This is how our ancestors have always done it'. This is because values are often used rhetorically and with rather conservative intentions designed to enhance professional tradition, authority and identity.

If we have shown nothing else here, we believe we have demonstrated that the view that professions are static and have stable values is illusory. While occupational groups and individual professionals may like to enhance their status, identity and significance by appealing to elements of tradition such as values, professions are in a constant state of flux and negotiation with a social context that is itself changing. Historically, professions have changed their ways of operating and conceiving of themselves in order to be perceived as relevant by the rest of society. The same process continues.

Professionals will change, and are changing, their espoused and enacted values, sometimes adopting new ones, sometimes emphasising particular values over others, always reinterpreting the meanings and understandings of their values. The relationship between values and professions is thus necessarily a living and lively one, though this is often not apparent to the casual observer at any particular moment in time. The dynamics of this relationship could be much better and more critically examined and understood both in terms of academic understanding and professional practice.

Such work could potentially yield significant knowledge about the identity, self-concept and nature of both professions and values, which would help us to understand much better what is expected and desired of professions both now and in the future. A better understanding of professional–value relations might be a kind of 'royal road' to seeing what the key issues surrounding professional work are in the contemporary world. This is not just a matter of academic interest; this kind of endeavour bears upon the expectations and trust that members of professional groups and members of society in general can hope to negotiate with each other.

Conflict, cost and negotiation

'Laminated' professional values may present themselves to practitioners and members of the public as uncontroversial, eternal, inevitable, set in stone. As we have seen constantly throughout this book, nothing could be further from reality. The identification, adoption, interpretation and enactment of values in professions is a highly temporal, social process, despite the fact that even the professions themselves may not always recognise this. Professional values come into being and are sustained by a complex and little examined process of negotiation within occupational groups and by those groups relating to wider society for a variety of ends. They are constructed in, and for, a particular context. Inevitably, there is a political aspect to this. Whose values will be adopted? Which values will become the 'official' values of the profession and who decides this? And whose interests and purposes will be served overtly, and covertly, by the values that are adopted?

Politics and negotiation also impinge upon the *enactment* of values in day-to-day professional work and behaviour. Individual professionals working in managed organisations have to negotiate the performance of their core professional values with others on a daily basis. Sometimes the cost of adhering to those values may be too high for the individuals concerned and fundamental compromises may have to be made. A number of examples in the previous chapters, from leisure managers to nurses, have revealed the quotidian politics of continuing to negotiate the maintenance and enactment of professional values.

This very practical aspect of maintaining standards and a sense of professional identity and responsibility is of vital importance in assessing the nature of professional work today. Yet perhaps it is too often underestimated. We expect much of professions and professionals with their high ideals and values expressed in codes and other documents. But perhaps we have not paid sufficient attention to the *realpolitik* of actual adherence to these in professional life. This is an important practical issue in the ongoing negotiation of the identity and place of professions and professionals in society, which requires attention if we are not to witness a collapse of trust in occupational groups which are much needed but little understood.

There can be no doubt that many professions *perceive* themselves as increasingly under attack, e.g. teachers, doctors and social workers. Whether or not there is a 'crisis' in the professions generally may be debatable, but there can be little doubt that professionals are increasingly coming under state regulation, being challenged by a better-educated and less deferential public, and under constant scrutiny by media ever interested in scandal and lapses from grace.

The ecology of professional–value relationships

One of the factors which has perhaps contributed to a lack of active interest in the relationship between values and professional practice may be a perception that the nature and functioning of professional values is a matter for professions themselves. An emergent insight from the contributions to this book is that professional values are to be seen as developing from, and acting within, a complex ecology of factors and pressures. Depending on the aspirations of occupational groups and individuals and social contextual factors such as organisational aims and structures, values may be adopted, adapted, discarded, reinterpreted, enacted or even completely ignored.

It may well suit both professions and the ordinary citizenry to behave as if professional values exist in a kind of pristine isolation from common social life. However, it is both more important and more interesting if the value–profession relationship is seen within an ecological perspective that properly recognises the wide range of factors that shape and maintain values in theory and in practice.

Different professions can exist in very different ecologies or contexts. Caring professions in public service may have different aims, aspirations, pressures, etc. from construction professions working mainly in the private sector, such as engineers. *Within* a particular sphere of activity, such as the caring professions, there can be considerable differences in the ideologies espoused by nurses, doctors and social workers, as illustrated in the contributions above. Moreover, within any one professional group there may also be differences in the values espoused and enacted in practice by professionals working in the public or private sector. A highly paid corporate lawyer working for a City firm is in a very different situation to the salaried lawyer who has chosen to work in a neighbourhood law centre. Similar contrasts can be easily imagined for doctors and teachers. These specific differences of ecology (or ecologies) need to be taken into account more in thinking about professions and values.

The need for critical awareness and curiosity

One of the most surprising, even disturbing, overall issues to arise out of this volume is the lack of critical awareness and curiosity about the nature of the relationship between professions and values. Indeed, this lack poses a challenging research question in its own right. Given the dynamic complexity of this relationship and its fundamental importance for professional identity, it might be expected that most, if not all, professionals and professional groups would be actively and continuously engaged in critically assessing their value base and interpreting this for practice. The chapters above suggest that mostly this does not occur. The legal profession, for example, which codifies, regulates and mediates values in its daily work, seems largely uninterested in articulating and criticising its own value base, allowing an informal value curriculum to shape the training of its entrants in ways that might be far from justifiable and desirable.

It is perhaps easier to speculate why practitioners might find constant interrogation of their values rather threatening and be happy to maintain a '*status quo*' rather than be seen as 'rocking the boat', particularly if they already perceive themselves as somewhat beleaguered. However, more poignantly, the academic community in its teaching and research consistently fails to examine the espoused and enacted values upon which it is based and which it may want to promote. This leaves it open to serving all manner of purposes, some of which may be distinctly dubious. Given that the study of values in professions is complex and fascinating, one might also hope that it would engage the best efforts of academics. The fact that it does not seems something of an indictment for researchers who claim to be interested in the critical evaluation of professions and practice in major spheres of social life.

It is safe to conclude on the basis of our explorations here that there is a desperate need for more critical curiosity and exploration of the relationship between values and professions. In the next section, we will make some suggestions as to how this might be taken forward by researchers and others interested in doing this.

What is to be done?

The relationship between values and professional practice is not significant just for professions and their members. Because of the importance of professional work and the values it embodies in society as a whole, this relationship must be of some significance to all the citizens who must put their trust and well-being in the hands of particular occupational groups (Fukuyama 1996; O'Neill 2002). Professional values are in a certain sense then 'everybody's business'. The insights emerging from the individual chapters in this book, and from the book as a whole, have considerable practical implications for a number of groups. These can be spelled out a bit more.

Professional bodies often have responsibility for codifying the values that their members are supposed to adopt and maintain and for maintaining compliance to them. It perhaps behoves them to think more critically and self-consciously about the process of articulating and adopting particular values. They might also like to become more involved in understanding just exactly what use is made of 'official' values in practice.

Perhaps more sophisticated, helpful and realistic approaches to incorporating values in practice can be developed if a more active and critical attitude is adopted to the whole issue of selecting and propagating values for particular professional groups. Most professions would probably benefit from involving members of the general public in their deliberations about the adoption and enactment of values. This would allow some sharing of responsibility and a wider perspective on which values really are important and realistic. They might also benefit from being less inward and looking at the ways that values are adopted and enacted in other professional groups, perhaps ones that are distant from their own.

At present, most professions tend to regard their values as their own exclusive concern and property, as if no other groups or individuals had a stake in them. Moreover, statements of values are often produced by the élite of the profession and are designed for public consumption only in the sense that they embody the claims for recognition and legitimisation by the wider society. Thus professions often claim to exist for the sake of protecting and serving their users. The exclusion of any input into such statements from the outside seems all the more anomalous, particularly when consumer responsiveness, effective governance and accountability are highly prized by the general public.

If professional values are everybody's business because of the impact of professions on most parts of life, then *ordinary citizens* may have an enhanced role and responsibility in the dialogue as to what values should be adopted and enacted. It is true, however, that currently neither the citizenry nor professional groups seem particularly keen to get lay involvement in discussion about professional values. It is also true that there could well be practical problems in recruiting people to take part. Are they to be invited, self-selected, or representative of wider society in some way? Still, the effort might be well worth making as the public is largely ignorant in regard to the ways in which values are espoused, expressed and mediated, and it is too easy for citizens to be negatively critical of professional attitudes and practices. This, in turn, can contribute to the demoralisation of professionals and erode trust in the work of people whose services are actually very much needed.

Perhaps there is a more constructive 'critical friend' role that might be adopted here that would allow members of the public to better understand value issues in professions and perhaps to directly contribute to the revision of these values. This might enhance service, trust and mutual appreciation rather than perpetuating ever-increasing dissatisfaction with the professions as the proverbial 'conspiracies against the laity'.

Individual professionals often give little thought to the importance of values in their work unless they are faced with some kind of direct dilemma which challenges their functioning, assumptions and identity. Here again, a more active approach to self-consciously understanding, adopting and interpreting values in the context of everyday practice might be interesting and invigorating, adding depth and an extra dimension of responsibility to work.

Unless individual professionals have a realistic and articulated understanding of the values that they work by, they are not in a strong position to criticise, defend or modify them, nor to discuss those values with interested others such a members of the public who use professional services. Developing a more critical understanding and approach to values in everyday professional practice might help professionals better comprehend and value their own roles. It might also help them to engage in more open and trusting relationships with clients, which would enhance the long-term confidence and value of their work.

Educators and trainers have a potentially vital role in enhancing the capacity of professions, individual professionals and members of the public in their selection and enactment of values. They can introduce the critical issues that we have discussed in this book and help people to identify and evaluate espoused and enacted values so that they are more likely to have their values than their values having them. Currently, as we have seen, teachers and trainers are just as likely as anyone else to have unexamined values. Furthermore, they may find themselves teaching abstractions about ethics, values and behaviour which are directly contradicted by the realities of life in professional practice, leaving learners open to the acquisition of an informal practical curriculum that might be antipathetic to official espoused professional values.

There is a lot of scope for teachers and trainers of professionals to become much more competent analysts of living values in the real world and then to help others gain analytic and critical techniques. To become more competent, however, they will probably need the best efforts of researchers looking much more closely at all aspects of the relationship between values and professional practice.

To return to a key theme of this chapter – the whole area of understanding the relationship between values, professions and values in different kinds of professional practice is not well understood. If practitioners, teachers, professional bodies and citizens are to become more sophisticated participants about the issues raised in this book, *researchers* of all kinds must become more involved in finding out more about how values are involved and function in different professions and professional contexts. While there has been much sociological work done on professions and upon some individual occupational groups and there has been philosophical scrutiny of values, relatively little has been done to explore the relationships between values and professional practice. It is to the agenda for research, then, that we now turn.

Directions for further research and enquiry

Given the limited attention to relationships between professions, professionals and values, there is enormous scope for further investigations in order to further practical and theoretical understanding and aid critique. Such research might range from clarification of language and concepts to empirical work on the analysis of values and meanings in particular contexts. Here are just a few ideas that might give some idea of the range, scope and type of approaches and methods that could be employed.

Comparative empirical sociological and organisational studies of different professions

Many professions deal with issues of values and practice as if they were their own exclusive preserve. There is much to be learned from the ways in which different kinds of professions in different contexts adopt and implement their values. What might caring professions in a public context learn from leisure-oriented professions, such as sport which is situated in the private sector? There is a lot of scope for more detailed studies of the evolution and use of values in individual professions and then for comparison between professional groups. One result of such studies might be to clarify whether there are certain values that are shared by all professions and, indeed, whether all professions can be partly defined by their adoption of particular values. A specific set of comparative studies that might be undertaken could also look at how different professional organisations actually establish their values. It would also be useful to understand how professional values are refracted and changed by different organisational contexts and aims in situations within the public and private sectors where professionals of different kinds mix together.

Users' perspectives on professions and their values

Precisely because many professions seem to regard the definition and implementation of formal values as a matter for autonomous organisational choice, it would be useful to know a good deal more about how *clients* might view professions and their values. Moreover, there is a case for examining *how* these values impact upon the users for whose benefit they are ostensibly in large part created. Another key question for investigation is exactly *who are the clients* for particular professions? One of the more striking things to emerge from some of the contributions is that there is not always a single person who is seeking the service/expert knowledge. Sometimes the client might be a firm or local or central government, raising the question of exactly how this difference is reflected in the ideology held by the professionals who are working in that particular context.

Having defined who exactly the users of the services are, one could then investigate what they notice about the values of the professions whose services they employ. What values do they think should be adopted and enacted? Such basic information, which could easily be obtained by empirical research, is largely lacking. It would be interesting in a pluralistic, egalitarian society to know whether attitudes of different social groups and types were the same or different. Do women, or members of ethnic minorities, or young people have different ideas about which values professionals should adopt and how they might be implemented in practice? Some work has already been done on this topic, particularly in the caring professions such as medicine and nursing, but it would be fascinating to have this information for a wider selection of professions.

Values in individual professional practice

A great deal more empirical work could also be done to find out just how exactly particular values, professional, personal and other, actually do work out in practice and in encounters with clients. Does it make any difference as to what values are adopted at a formal organisational level to the way in which individual practitioners conduct their work? What sort of difference might this be? Here again, inter-professional comparative empirical research might reveal much about the similarities and differences between organisations and individual practice.

Analysing teaching and training in professional values

As we have seen, professional socialisation and education is a vital part of understanding the nature, place and operationalisation of values in professional practice. Presently, little is known of the intended and unintended effects of different kinds of educational and training experience and methods in instilling values in practitioners. The pedagogical strategies used need to be much better understood and more investigation needs to take place into the impact of theoretical and experiential learning, formal and informal, upon the values of initiates into professions. Perhaps some ethnographical work upon students in different professions undertaking education and training would be useful here. Again, there are some pioneering studies in medicine, nursing and law.

Conceptualising and arguing about values and understandings of professionalism more adequately

In *Professionalism: the third logic*, Friedson, one of the earliest sociological critical analysts of professions and professionalism, notes the need for a better conceptual understanding of the nature and place of professions and professionalism in society to complement the logics of the market and consumerism on the one hand and the firm or bureacracy on the other. Friedson suggests that professions have not defended themselves adequately amidst pressures coming from both these sources. He writes:

> When they do defend themselves they rely primarily on a rhetoric of good intentions which is belied by the patently self-interested character of many of their activities. What they almost never do is spell out the principles underlying the institutions that organize and support the way they do their work and take active responsibility for their organization.
>
> (Friedson 2001: 3)

He goes on to to advocate the need for a new, third logic that can support profesional identity and activity:

> I hold that a logical model [of professionalism] based on a theoretically chosen foundation can provide focus and direction to empirical studies, at the very least by serving as a clear target for criticism and revision.
>
> (Friedson 2001: 5)

The import of Friedson's comment is that not all the research that might be undertaken into values in professional practice needs to be empirically based. Part of what makes it difficult to research the relations between professions and values is lack of conceptual clarity as to what is being looked at.

So there is an important job for conceptual researchers such as philosophers in helping to clarify the nature of professions and values which needs to carried on simultaneously with empirical work. Conceptual and empirical work combined may lead to some striking new insights into the nature of professions and that of values. This may have wide social and intellectual implications in helping professions reconceptualise themselves and engage with the public. A further conceptual task that might be undertaken is to analyse understandings among the general public and particular professional groups as to what is understood by the ideal of 'the good professional'. This would clarify an idea which is presently little understood in either general or specific terms.

Understanding and determining the context and role of professions and their values

Social analysts and policy makers might perhaps give more analytic attention to the context and role of professions and their values in wider society.

At the moment, professions and professionals are lauded by some, distrusted by others. There may be a crisis in professional identity and authority partly fuelled by a loss of trust in particular occupational groups on the part of a questioning, consumerist public. There is thus a considerable need for some critical and speculative analytic thinking about the place and future of professions, professionals and professionalism in advanced Western society. Inevitably, this will involve consideration of the normative and enacted values that professions should adopt.

Conclusion

Many of us regard ourselves as professionals. All of us use the services of professionals. So the way in which professionals adopt and enact their values in practice is of importance to us all on a day-to-day basis.

In this book, we have begun to show that the relationship between values, professions and professional practice is an integral, complex and, above all, fascinating one. You cannot have a profession without values, even if you do not appreciate the values that are either adopted by an occupational group or enacted by its members. Given the fundamental importance of values for establishing professional identity and assuring public trust, it is surprising that so little attention has been paid to this topic. It is our hope that by selectively looking at some aspects of this relationship from a variety of analytic perspectives, focusing on a limited number of professions, some of which are quite differently contextualised and constituted from others, we will have made the case for much more attention to be focused on this area in future.

In a short book, we have not been able to look at more than a small segment of all possible professions. We are acutely aware that there are many other occupational groups and individuals that are either candidates for professional designation or see themselves as fleeing this kind of description which might have been considered – for example, school teachers, accountants and the police. Equally, we are conscious that this book has been biased towards the consideration of values and professional practice within the context of the public, as opposed to the private, sector. Nonetheless, we hope that enough different approaches and questions have been raised to engender more general interest in this topic area in the future. The relationship between professions, professional practice and values is everybody's business in advanced Western societies. It is time that this was much more firmly reflected in academic as well as practitioner agendas.

Bibliography

Aaron H, Mann T and Taylor T (1994) (eds) *Values and Public Policy*. The Brookings Institution, Washington, DC.

Abbott A (1988) *The System of Professions: an essay on the division of expert labour*. University of Chicago Press, Chicago.

ACLEC (1996) *First Report on Legal Education and Training*. The Lord Chancellor's Advisory Committee on Legal Education and Conduct, www.ukcle.ac.uk/resources/aclec.html

Addison J (2000) On the pleasures of the imagination. In: C Harrison, P Wood and J Gaiger (eds) *Art in Theory, 1648–1815*. Blackwell, Oxford.

Albrecht GL, Fitzpatrick R and Scrimshaw SC (eds) (2000) Introduction. *The Handbook of Social Studies in Health and Medicine*. Sage Publications, London.

Alimo-Metcalfe B and Alban-Metcalfe J (2002) Half the battle. *Health Service Journal*. 112 (5795): 26–7.

Allen D (2000) Faculty practice: a model to bridge the theory–practice divide. *British Journal of Community Nursing*. 5 (10): 504–10.

Allen D (2001) *The Changing Shape of Nursing Practice: the role of nurses in the hospital division of labour*. Routledge, London.

Allmendinger P (1998) Planning practice and the post-modern debate. *International Planning Studies*. 3 (2): 227–48.

Armstrong D (2000) Social theorising about health and illness. In: GL Albrecht, R Fitzpatrick and SC Scrimshaw (eds) *The Handbook of Social Studies in Health and Medicine*. Sage Publications, London.

Armstrong J, Dixon R and Robinson S (1999) *The Decision Makers: ethics for engineers*. Thomas Telford Publishing, London.

Association of Social Anthropologists of the UK and the Commonwealth (2003) *Ethical Guidelines for Good Research Practice*, http://les1.man.ac.uk/asa/Ethics/ethics.htm

Atkinson P (1984) Training for certainty. *Social Science and Medicine*. 19: 949–56.

Avis M (1999) Social justice and the right to health care. In: J Robinson, M Avis, J Latimer *et al.* (eds) *Interdisciplinary Perspectives on Health Policy and Practice*. Churchill Livingstone, Edinburgh.

Avis P (1989) *Anglicanism and the Christian Church*. T and T Clark, Edinburgh.

Banks S (1995) *Ethics and Values in Social Work*. BASW/Macmillan, London.

Barker P, Jackson S and Stevenson C (1999) The need for psychiatric nursing: towards a multidimensional theory of caring. *Nursing Inquiry*. 6: 103–11.

Barker PJ, Reynolds W and Stevenson C (1997) The human science basis of psychiatric nursing: theory and practice. *Journal of Advanced Nursing.* **25**: 660–7.

Baum H (1997) Teaching practice. *Journal of Planning Education and Research.* 17: 21–29.

Bayles M (1981) *Professional Ethics.* Wadsworth Publishing, Belmount, CA.

Becker H (1970a) The nature of a profession. In: H Becker (ed) *Sociological Work: method and substance.* Aldine Publishing Company, Chicago, IL.

Becker H (1970b) Whose side are we on? In: H Becker (ed) *Sociological Work: method and substance.* Aldine Publishing Company, Chicago, IL.

Becker HS, Greer B, Hughes E *et al.* (1961) *Boys in White: student culture in medical school.* University of Chicago Press, Chicago, IL.

Bennion AR (1969) *Professional Ethics.* Charles Knight, London.

Berns S (1993) *Concise Jurisprudence.* The Federation Press, Sydney.

Black N (2002) Preface. In: A-M Rafferty and M Traynor (eds) *Exemplary Research for Nursing and Midwifery.* Routledge, London.

Blake W (1975) Marginal notes to Reynolds' *Discourses.* In: J Reynolds *Discourses on Art.* Yale University Press, New Haven, CT.

Bligh J (2001) Assessment: the gap between theory and practice. *Medical Education.* **35** (4): 312.

Blom Cooper L (1985) *A Child in Trust.* London Borough of Brent, London.

Bocock R and Thompson K (1985) *Religion and Ideology.* Manchester University Press, Manchester.

Bottomley A (1996) (ed) *Feminist Perspectives on the Foundational Subjects of Law.* Cavendish, London.

Brandt RB (1992) *Morality, Utilitarianism and Rights.* Cambridge University Press, Cambridge.

Braye S and Preston-Shoot M (1998) Social work and the law. In: R Adams, L Dominelli and M Payne (eds) *Social Work: themes issues and critical debates.* Macmillan, Basingstoke.

Brint S (1994) *In an Age of Experts: the changing role of professionals in politics and public life.* Princeton University Press, Princeton, NJ.

British Association of Social Workers (2002) *The Code of Ethics for Social Work.* BASW, London.

British Sociological Association (2003). http:// www.britsoc.uk/bsa

Broadbent J, Dietrich M and Roberts J (1997) *The End of Professions? The restructuring of professional work.* Routledge, London.

Bruce S (1996) *Religion in the Modern World: from cathedrals to cults.* Oxford University Press, Oxford.

Bruhl E (1996) Book review of Patricia Williams' *The Rooster's Egg: on the persistence of prejudice. Michigan Law Review.* **94** (6): 2009–15.

Budd M (1996) *Values of Art: pictures, poetry and music.* Penguin, London.

Butcher H (1994) The concept of community practice. In: L Haywood and H Butcher (eds) *Community Leisure and Recreation.* Heinemann, London.

Butler BC (1981) *The Theology of Vatican II.* Darton, Longman and Todd, London.

Butler-Sloss E (1988) *Report of the Inquiry into Child Abuse in Cleveland.* Cm. 412. HMSO, London.

Cantwell Smith W (1993) *What is Scripture?* SCM Press, London.

Carper B (1978) Fundamental patterns of knowing in nursing. *Advances in Nursing Science.* **1** (1): 13–23.

Carr-Saunders AM and Wilson PA (1933) *The Professions.* Frank Cass, London.

Central Council for Education and Training in Social Work (CCETSW) (1995) *Assuring Quality in Social Work* – 1. Rules and Requirements for the Diploma in Social Work. CCETSW, London.

Chadwick R (ed) (1994) *Ethics in the Professions.* Avebury, Aldershot.

Church Information Office (1985) *Faith in the City: a call for action by church and nation.* The Archbishop of Canterbury's Commission on Urban Priority Areas, Church Publishing House, London.

Church Information Office (1990) *Faith in the Countryside.* The Archbishop of Canterbury's Commission on Rural Affairs, Churchman Publishing, London.

Claringbull D (1994) *Ministry in the Market Place.* Canterbury Press, Norwich.

Clark C (2000) *Social Work Ethics.* Palgrave, Basingstoke.

Coalter F (1998) Leisure studies, leisure policy and social citizenship: the failure or the limits of welfare. *Leisure Studies.* **17** (1): 21–36.

Coate MA (1989) *Clergy Stress: the hidden conflicts in ministry.* Society for Promoting Christian Knowledge, London.

Coburn D and Willis E (2000) The medical profession: knowledge, power and autonomy. In: GL Albrecht, R Fitzpatrick and S Scrimshaw (eds) *Handbook of Social Studies in Health and Medicine.* Sage Publications Ltd, London.

Cole A (1991) Upholding the code. *Nursing Times.* **87** (27): 26–9.

Cole A (2002a) Walking tall. *Health Service Journal.* **112** (5815): 24–7.

Cole A (2002b) Further to fall. *Health Service Journal.* **112** (5809): 28–31.

Cole B (2000) *Trends in the Solicitors' Profession – Annual Statistics Report.* Law Society, London.

Collier R (1991) Masculinism, law and law teaching. *International Journal of the Sociology of Law.* **19**: 427–51.

Commission on Faith and Order (1982) *Baptism, Eucharist and Ministry.* World Council of Churches, Geneva.

Committee on Publication Ethics (1999) *The COPE Report.* British Medical Journal Bookshop, London.

Conaghan J (1996) Tort law and the feminist critique of reason. In: A Bottomley (ed) *Feminist Perspectives on the Foundational Subjects of Law.* Cavendish, London.

Corlett J, Palfreyman JW, Staines HJ *et al.* (2003) Factors influencing theoretical knowledge and practical skill acquisition in student nurses: an empirical experiment. *Nurse Education Today.* **23** (3): 183–9.

Cowley S (1999) Nursing in a managerial age. In: I Norman and S Cowley (eds) *The Changing Nature of Nursing in a Managerial Age.* Blackwell Science, Oxford.

Crisp R and Slote M (eds) (1997) *Virtue Ethics.* Oxford University Press, Oxford.

Croft S (1999) *Ministry in Three Dimensions.* Darton, Longman and Todd, London.

Crompton JL and Wicks BE (1986) Citizen and administrator perspectives of equity in the delivery of park services. *Leisure Sciences.* **8** (4): 341–65.

Crompton JL and Wicks BE (1990) Predicting the equity preferences of park and recreation services. *Journal of Leisure Research.* **22** (1): 18–35.

Cutcliffe J and Goward P (2000) Mental health nurses and qualitative research methods: a mutual attraction? *Journal of Advanced Nursing.* **31** (3): 590–98.

Dale R (1976) Work, culture and consciousness. *People and Work, Unit 9.* Open University Press, Milton Keynes.

Davie G (1994) *Religion in Britain since 1945.* Blackwell, Oxford.

Davie G (2000) *Religion in Modern Europe: a memory mutates.* Oxford University Press, Oxford.

Davies J (2001) Rules of engagement. *Health Service Journal.* **111** (5773): 22–5.

Davis M (1996) Some paradoxes of whistle-blowing. *Business and Professional Ethics Journal.* **15** (1): 3–21.

Dawn M and Peterson E (2000) *The Unnecessary Pastor.* Eeerdmans, Grand Rapids, MI.

Dawson S, Mole V, Winstanley D and Sherval J (1995) *Managing in the NHS: a study of senior managers.* HMSO, London.

Day RO (1979) *The English Clergy, 1558–1642.* Leicester University Press, Leicester.

Department of Health (1995) *Messages from Research* HMSO, London.

Department of Health (2000a) *Framework for the Assessment of Children in Need and their Families.* HMSO, London.

Department of Health (2000b) *The NHS Plan.* Cm. 4818. HMSO, London.

Department of Health (2001) *Shifting the Balance.* Department of Health, London.

Department of Health (2002) *Code of Conduct for NHS Managers.* Department of Health, London.

Department of Health and Social Security (1983) *The NHS Management Inquiry.* Department of Health and Social Security, London.

Department of Health, Home Office and Department for Education and Employment (1999) *Working Together to Safeguard Children.* HMSO, London.

Dubos R (1960) *Mirage of Health.* Unwin, London.

Dunne J (1993) *Back to the Rough Ground.* University of Notre Dame Press, Notre Dame, IN.

Dunstan GR (1967) The Sacred Ministry as a Profession. *Theology.* **70** (568): 433–42.

The Economist (2003) Government and the market send out mixed signals to the universities. 26 July: 33.

Edgar A (2003) How effective are codes of nursing ethics? In: W Tadd (ed) *Ethical and Professional Issues in Nursing.* Palgrave Macmillan, Basingstoke.

Elston M (1991) The politics of professional power: medicine in a changing health service. In: J Gabe, M Calnan and M Bury (eds) *The Sociology of the Health Service.* Routledge, London.

Etzioni A (1995a) *The Spirit of Community.* Fontana Press, London.

Etzioni A (ed) (1995b) *New Communitarian Thinking.* University Press of Virginia, Charlottesville.

European Council of Nursing (2002) *European Codes of Conduct in Nursing: report of Work Package 2*. ECN, University of Maastricht, Maastricht.

Faber H (1971) *Pastoral Care in the Modern Hospital*. SCM Press, London.

Finley L (1993) Breaking women's silence in law: the dilemma of the gendered nature of legal reasoning. In: P Smith (ed) *Feminist Jurisprudence*. Oxford University Press, New York.

Flannery A (1981) *Vatican Council II: the conciliar and post-conciliar documents*. Fowler Wright Books, Leominster.

Foot P (1978) *Virtues and Vices and Other Essays in Moral Philosophy*. Blackwell, Oxford.

Forester J (1993) Learning from practice stories: the priority of practical judgement. In: F Fischer and J Forester (eds) *The Argumentative Turn in Policy Analysis and Planning*. University College London Press, London.

Friedson E (1970) *Profession of Medicine*. Dodd Mead, New York.

Friedson E (2001) *Professionalism: the third logic*. Polity Press, Cambridge.

Fukuyama F (1996) *Trust: the social virtues and the creation of prosperity*. Penguin Books, London.

Gardiner P (2003) A virtue ethics approach to moral dilemmas in medicine. *Journal of Medical Ethics*. **29** (5): 5, 297–302.

General Social Care Council (2002) *Codes of Practice for Social Care Workers and Employers*. General Social Care Council, London.

Good B (1994) *Medicine, Rationality and Experience: an anthropological perspective*. Cambridge University Press, Cambridge.

Goodin RE (1991) Utility and the good. In: P Singer (ed) *A Companion to Ethics*. Blackwell, Oxford.

Gould N (1996) Using imagery in reflective learning. In: N Gould and I Taylor (eds) *Reflective Learning for Social Work*. Arena, Aldershot.

Gournay K (1999) The future of nursing research will be better served by a shift to quantitative methodologies. *Clinical Effectiveness in Nursing*. **3**: 1–3.

Gournay K (2003) Drug treatments for schizophrenia: why they offer the only hope for patients. *Mental Health Practice*. **6** (6): 16–17.

Gournay K and Brooking J (1994) Community psychiatric nurses in primary health care. *British Journal of Psychiatry*. **165**: 231–8.

Greaves D (1996) Concepts of health, illness and disease. In: D Greaves and H Upton (eds) *Philosophical problems in health care*. Avebury, Aldershot.

Greenwood E (1957) Attributes of a profession. *Social Work*. **2** (3): 45–55.

Grice P (2001) *The Conception of Value*. Oxford University Press, Oxford.

Griffith JAG (1997) *The Politics of the Judiciary*. (5e). Fontana Press, London.

Grimshaw JM, Eccles MP, Walker AE *et al.* (2002) Changing physicians' behaviour: what works and thoughts on getting more things to work. *Journal of Continuing Education for Health Professionals*. **22** (4): 237–43.

Gula RM (1996) *Ethics in Pastoral Ministry*. Paulist Press, Mahwah, NJ.

Habermas J (1989) *The Structural Transformation of the Public Sphere*. Massachusetts Institute of Technology Press, Cambridge MA.

Hague E, Thomas C and Williams S (2000) Equity or exclusion? Contemporary experiences in post-industrial urban leisure. In: *Just Leisure*. Leisure Studies Association Publication No. 72, Brighton.

Hall C and Hanniford R (eds) (1996) *Order and Ministry*. Gracewing, Leominster.

Hammersley M (1989) *The Dilemma of Qualitative Method: Herbert Blumer and the Chicago School*. Routledge, London.

Hare P (2003) The UK's Research Assessment Exercise: impact on institutions, departments and individuals. *Higher Education Management and Policy*. **15** (1): 23–36.

Harley S (2002) The impact of research selectivity on academic work and identity in UK universities. *Studies in Higher Education*. **27** (2): 187–205.

Harrison C, Wood P and Gaiger J (eds) (2000) *Art in Theory, 1648–1815*. Blackwell, Oxford.

Harrison S, Hunter DJ, Marnoch G and Pollitt C (1992) *Just Managing: power and culture in the National Health Service*. Macmillan, Basingstoke.

Hastings A (1987) *A History of the English Church*. Society for Promoting Christian Knowledge, London.

Hastings A (1991) *Modern Catholicism: Vatican II and after*. Society for Promoting Christian Knowledge, London.

Hauerwas S (1981) *A Community of Character*. University of Notre Dame Press, Notre Dame, IN.

Her Majesty's Stationery Office (2001) *Learning from Bristol: the report of the public inquiry into children's heart surgery at the Bristol Royal Infirmary, 1984–1995*. HMSO, London.

Higher Education Funding Council for England (2001) *Research in Nursing and Allied Health Professions: report of the Task Group 3 to HEFCE and the Department of Health*. Higher Education Funding Council for England, London.

Howell S and McNamee MJ (2003) Local justice and public sector leisure policy. *Leisure Studies*. **22** (1): 17–35.

Hume D (1996) Of the standard of taste. In: D Hume (ed) *Essays*. Oxford University Press, Oxford.

Hunt G (1994) New professionals? New ethics? In: G Hunt and P Wainwright (eds) *Expanding the Role of the Nurse*. Blackwell Scientific, Oxford.

Hunt G (1995) *Whistle-blowing in the NHS*. Edward Arnold, London.

Hunt SJ (2002) *Religion in Western Society*. Palgrave, Basingstoke.

Hussey T (1996) Nursing ethics and codes of professional conduct. *Nursing Ethics*. **3** (3): 250–8.

Illich I (1976) *Limits to Medicine*. Marion Boyars, London.

Institution of Civil Engineers (2001) *Royal Charter, By-laws, Regulations and Rules*. Institution of Civil Engineers, London.

Ireland P (2002) History, critical legal studies and the mysterious disappearance of capitalism. *Modern Law Review*. **65** (1): 106–19.

Irvine D (1997) The performance of doctors (i): professionalism and self regulation in a changing world. *British Medical Journal*. **314**: 1540.

Jewson N (1976) The disappearance of the sick man from medical cosmology, 1770–1870. *Sociology.* **10**: 225–44.

Keep J and McClenahan J (2002) Organisational values: a case study in the NHS. In: B New and J Neuberger (eds) *Hidden Assets: values and decision-making in the NHS.* King's Fund, London.

Kennedy D (1982) Legal education as training for hierarchy. In: D Kairys (ed) *The Politics of Law: a progressive critique.* Pantheon Books, New York.

Koehn D (1994) Th*e Ground of Professional Ethics.* Routledge, London.

Laming Report (2003) *The Victoria Climbie Inquiry.* Report of an Inquiry by Lord Laming Cm. 5730.

Larkin GV (1993) Continuity in change: medical dominance in the United Kingdom. In: FW Hafferty and JB McKinlay (eds) *The Changing Medical Profession.* Oxford University Press, Oxford.

Larson MS (1977) *The Rise of Professionalism.* University of California Press, Berkeley, CA.

Lebacqz K (1985) *Professional Ethics: power and paradox.* Abingdon, Nashville, Tennessee.

Lineberry RL (1977) *Equality and Urban Policy: the distribution of municipal public service.* Sage, London.

Little J (1994) *Gender, Policy Processes and Planning.* Pergamon, Oxford.

Loftman P and Beazley M (1998) *Race Equality and Planning.* Local Government Association, London.

Lo Piccolo F and Thomas H (2001) Legal discourse, the individual and the claim for equality in planning. *Planning Theory and Practice.* **2** (2): 187–201.

Lyon D (1985) *The Steeple's Shadow.* Society for Promoting Christian Knowledge, London.

Macdonald KM (1995) *The Sociology of the Professions.* Sage Publications, London.

MacIntyre A (1981) *After Virtue* (1e). Duckworth, London.

Mackie J (1977) *Ethics: inventing right and wrong.* Penguin, Harmondsworth.

Malby B and Pattison S (1999) *Living Values in the NHS.* King's Fund, London.

Mansell W, Meteyard B and Thomson Λ (1995) *A Critical Introduction to Law.* Cavendish, London.

May T (2001) *Social Research* (3e). Open University Press, Buckingham and Philadelphia.

McGlynn C (1999) Women, representation and the legal academy. *Legal Studies.* **19**: 68–92.

McGuire MB (1987) *Religion: the social context.* Wadsworth, Belmont.

McKenna H (1997) *Nursing Theories and Models.* Routledge, London.

McKinlay JB and Stoeckle JD (1988) Corporatisation and the social transformation of doctoring. *Health Services.* **18**: 191–205.

McLoughlin JB (1973) *Control and Urban Planning.* Faber, London.

McNamee M (1994) Valuing leisure practice: towards a theoretical framework. *Leisure Studies.* **13** (1): 288–309.

McNamee MJ, Sheridan H and Buswell J (2000) Paternalism, professionalism and public sector leisure provision: the boundaries of a leisure profession. *Leisure Studies*. **19**: 199–209.

Melinsky H (1992) *The Shape of the Ministry*. Canterbury Press, Norwich.

Midgely M (2001) *Science and Poetry*. Routledge, London.

Miller DF and Hersen M (eds) (1992) *Research Fraud in the Behavioural and Biomedical sciences*. John Wiley & Sons, New York.

Minow M (1991) *Making All the Difference: inclusion, exclusion and American law*. Cornell University Press, Ithaca and London.

Moran J (2002) *Interdisciplinarity*. Routledge, London.

Morgan W (1994) *Leftist Theories of Sport*. University of Chicago Press, Chicago.

Neill S (1977) *Anglicanism*. Mowbrays, London.

Nelson RL and Trubeck DM (1992) New problems and new paradigms in studies of the legal profession. In: RL Nelson, DM Trubeck and RL Solomon (eds) *Lawyers' Ideals/Lawyers' Practices*. Cornell University Press, Ithaca and London.

New B (2002) Thinking about values. In: B New and J Neuberger (eds) *Hidden Assets: values and decision-making in the NHS*. King's Fund, London.

Nicholson D (1991) Planners' skills and planning practice. In: H Thomas and P Healey (eds) *Dilemmas of Planning Practice*. Avebury, Aldershot.

Nicolson D (1995) Telling tales: gender discrimination, gender construction and battered women who kill. *Feminist Legal Studies*. **2**(3): 185–206.

Noddings N (1984) *Caring: a feminine approach to ethics and moral education*. University of California, Berkeley, CA.

Nursing and Midwifery Council (2002a) *Code of Professional Conduct*. NMC, London.

Nursing and Midwifery Council (2002b) *Statistical Analysis of the Register, 1 April 2001 to 31 March 2002*. NMC, London.

Oakley A (1980) *Women Confined: towards a sociology of childbirth*. Martin Robertson, Oxford.

Oakley A (2000) *Experiments in Knowing: gender and method in the social sciences*. Polity Press, Cambridge.

O'Neill O (2002) *A Question of Trust*. Cambridge University Press, Cambridge.

Orchard H (2001) *Spirituality in Healthcare Communities*. Jessica Kingsley, London.

Parsons G (2002) *Perspectives on Civil Religion*. Ashgate, Aldershot.

Parsons T (1951) *The Social System*. Free Press, New York.

Parton N (2001) Risk and professional judgement. In: L Cull and J Roche (eds) *The Law and Social Work: contemporary issues for practice*. Palgrave, Basingstoke.

Paton R (1997) The trouble with values. Unpublished paper.

Pattison S (1989) *Alive and Kicking: towards a practical theology of illness and healing*. SCM Press, London.

Pattison S (1997) *The Faith of the Managers*. Cassell, London.

Pattison S (2000) Some objections to aims and objectives. In: GR Evans and M Percy (eds) *Managing the Church?* Sheffield Academic Press, Sheffield.

Pattison S (2001) Are nursing codes ethical? *Nursing Ethics*. **8** (1): 5–18.

Payne M (2002) Social work theories and reflective practice. In: R Adams, L Dominelli and M Payne (eds) *Social Work: themes issues and critical debates*. Macmillan, Basingstoke.

Pence G (1991) Virtue theory. In: P Singer (ed) *A Companion to Ethics*. Blackwell, Oxford.

Pickstone J (2000) *Ways of Knowing: a new history of science, technology and medicine*. Manchester University Press, Manchester.

Pink G, http://www.freedomtocare.org/page73.htm

Pithouse A (1994) The happy family: learning colleagueship in a social work team. In: A Coffey and P Atkinson (eds) *Occupational Socialization and Working Lives*. Ashgate, Aldershot.

Porter R (1997) *The Greatest Benefit to Mankind: a medical history of humanity from antiquity to the present*. Harper Collins, London.

Power M (1997) *The Audit Society: rituals of verification*. Oxford University Press, Oxford.

Rackley E (1997) Legal education and the illusion of law's objectivity. Undergraduate Dissertation, Cardiff Law School.

Ramsay AM (1985) *The Christian Priest Today*. Society for Promoting Christian Knowledge, London.

Ranson S, Bryman A and Hinnings B (1977) *Clergy, Ministers and Priests*. Routledge and Kegan Paul, London.

Reade E *(1987) British Town and Country Planning*. Open University Press, Milton Keynes.

Reason P (1994) *Participation in Human Inquiry*. Sage Publications, London.

Reynolds J (1975) *Discourses on Art*. Yale University Press, New Haven, CT.

Reynolds J (2000) Letters to *The Idler*. In: C Harrison, P Wood and J Gaiger (eds) *Art in Theory, 1648–1815*. Blackwell, Oxford.

Richardson J (2000a) Essay on the theory of painting. In: C Harrison, P Wood and J Gaiger (eds) *Art in Theory, 1648–1815*. Blackwell, Oxford.

Richardson J (2000b) The science of a connoisseur. In: C Harrison, P Wood and J Gaiger (eds) *Art in Theory, 1648–1815*. Blackwell, Oxford.

Russell A (1980) *The Clerical Profession*. Society for Promoting Christian Knowledge, London.

Salmon JW (1994) *The Corporate Transformation of Health Care*. Baywood, New York.

Salvage J (1990) The theory and practice of the 'new nursing'. *Nursing Times*. **86** (1): 42–5.

Sassi F (2003) Setting priorities for the evaluation of health interventions: when theory does not meet practice. *Health Policy*. **63** (2): 141–54.

Schimmel S (1997) *The Seven Deadly Sins*. Oxford University Press, Oxford.

Schon D (1984) *The Reflective Practitioner: how professionals think in action*. Basic Books, New York.

Scottish Executive (2003) *The Framework for Social Work Education in Scotland*. Scottish Executive, Edinburgh.

Shardlow SM (1998) Values, ethics and social work. In: R Adams, L Domenelli and M Payne (eds) *Social Work: themes, issues and critical debates.* Macmillan, Basingstoke.

Shaw GB (1946) *The Doctor's Dilemma.* Penguin Books, New York.

Sinclair S (1997) *Making Doctors: an institutional apprenticeship.* Berg, Oxford.

Smith C (1997) Children's Rights: have carers abandoned values? *Children and Society.* **11**: 3–15.

Snell J (2000) The short goodbye. *Health Service Journal.* **110** (5708): 24–7.

Solomon RC (1993) *Ethics and Excellence.* Oxford University Press, Oxford.

Spurgeon P and Barwell F (2002) The morale majority. *Health Service Journal.* **112** (5808): 22–4.

Stewart R, Blake J, Smith P and Wingate P (1980) *The District Administrator in the National Health Service.* King's Fund, London.

Stivers R (2001) *Technology as Magic: the triumph of the irrational.* Continuum, New York.

Sugarman D (1991) A hatred of disorder: legal science, liberalism and imperialism. In: P Fitzpatrick (ed) *Dangerous Supplements: resistance and renewal in jurisprudence.* Pluto Press, London.

Sykes S, Barty J and Knight J (1998) *The Study of Anglicanism.* T and T Clark, Edinburgh.

Tadd V (1994) Professional codes: an exercise in tokenism? *Nursing Ethics.* **1** (1): 15–23.

Talbot M (2000) *Make your Mission Statement Work.* How to Books Ltd, Oxford.

Thomas H (1980) The education of British town planners, 1965–1975. *Planning and Administration.* **7** (2): 67–78.

Thomas H (2000) *Race and Planning.* University College London Press, London.

Thomson A (1987) Critical legal education in Britain. *Journal of Law and Society.* **14** (1): 183–97.

Towler R and Coxon APM (1979) *The Fate of the Anglican Clergy.* Macmillan Press, London.

Tschudin V (1992) *Values.* Balliere Tindall, London.

Turner BS (2000) The history of the changing concepts of health and illness: outline of a general model of illness categories. In: GL Albrecht, R Fitzpatrick and SC Scrimshaw (eds) *The Handbook of Social Studies in Health and Medicine.* Sage Publications, London.

Unger RM (1986) *The Critical Legal Studies Movement.* Harvard University Press, Cambridge, MA and London.

United Kingdom Central Council for Nursing, Midwifery and Health Visiting (1986) *Project 2000: a new preparation for practice.* UKCC, London.

United Kingdom Central Council for Nursing, Midwifery and Health Visiting (1992) *The United Kingdom Central Council for Nursing, Midwifery and Health Visiting Code of Professional Conduct.* UKCC, London.

United Kingdom Central Council for Nursing, Midwifery and Health Visiting (1999) *Fitness for practice: the UKCC Commission for Nursing and Midwifery Education* (Chair: Sir Leonard Peach). UKCC, London.

Vernon S, Harris R ,and Ball C (1990) *Towards Social Work Law: legally competent professional practice.* Paper 4.2. Central Council for Education and Training in Social Work, London.

Wall A (1999) *Icebergs and Deckchairs: organisational change in the NHS.* Nuffield Trust, London.

Wall A (2001) *Being a Health Service Manager – Expectations and Experience: a study of four generations of managers in the NHS.* Nuffield Trust, London.

Walshe K and Smith J (2001) Cause and effect. *Health Service Journal.* **111** (5776): 20–3.

Watson G (1988) *The Civils: the story of the Institution of Civil Engineers.* Thomas Telford, London.

Watts T, Jones M, Wainwright P *et al.* (2002) Methodologies analysing individual practice in health care: a systematic review. *Journal of Advanced Nursing.* **35** (2): 238–56.

Weist WE and Smith EA (1990) *Ethics in Ministry.* Fortress Press, Minneapolis, MN.

Wells C (2002) Women law professors: negotiating and transcending gender identities at work. *Feminist Legal Studies.* **10** (1): 1–38.

Whipp M (1997) A healthy sense of vocation? *Contact.* **122**: 3–10.

Wilensky HL (1964) The professionalisation of everyone? *American Journal of Sociology.* **70**: 137–58.

Williams G (1982) *Learning the Law* (11e) Stevens and Sons, London.

Williams P (1991) *The Alchemy of Race and Rights: diary of a law school professor.* Harvard University Press, Cambridge, MA.

Wind JP, Burk JR, Comensch PF *et al.* (1991) *Clergy Ethics in a Changing Society.* Westminster/John Knox, Philadelphia, PA.

Index